D1232794

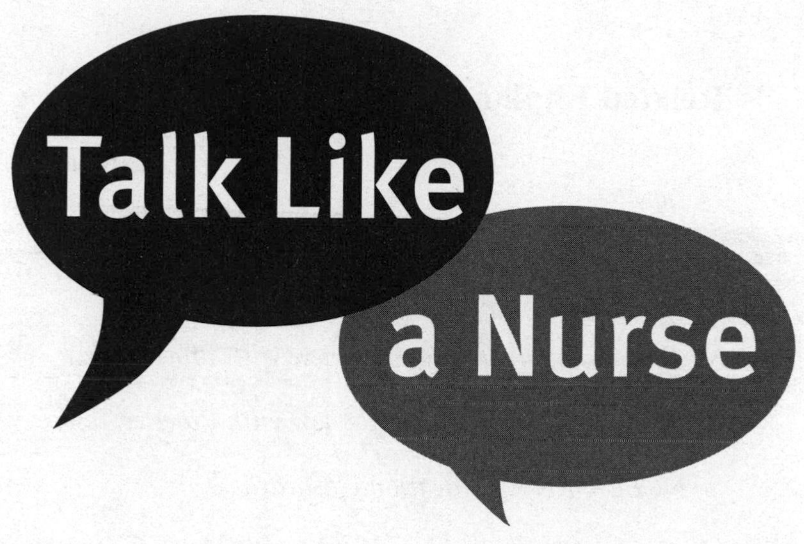
Talk Like
a Nurse

Related Kaplan Titles for Nurses

Test Preparation

NCLEX-RN® Premier with 2 Practice Tests

NCLEX-RN® Strategies, Practice, and Review with Practice Test

NCLEX-PN® Strategies, Practice, and Review with Practice Test

NCLEX-RN® Medication Flashcards

NCLEX-RN® Drug Guide: 300 Medications You Need to Know for the Exam

Nursing School Entrance Exams

CCRN®: Certification for Adult Critical Care Nurses

Career

Math for Nurses

Medical Terms for Nurses

Spanish for Nurses

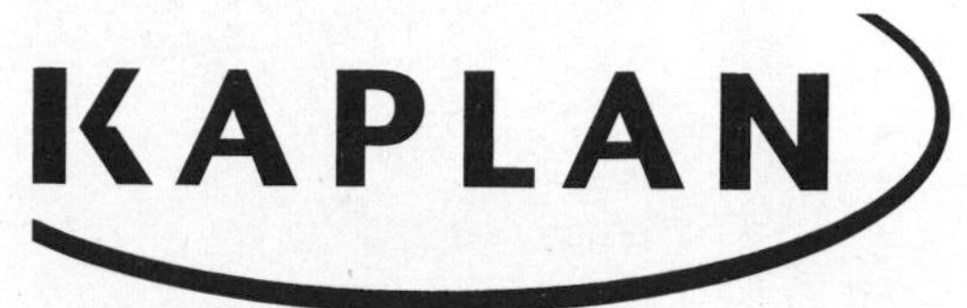

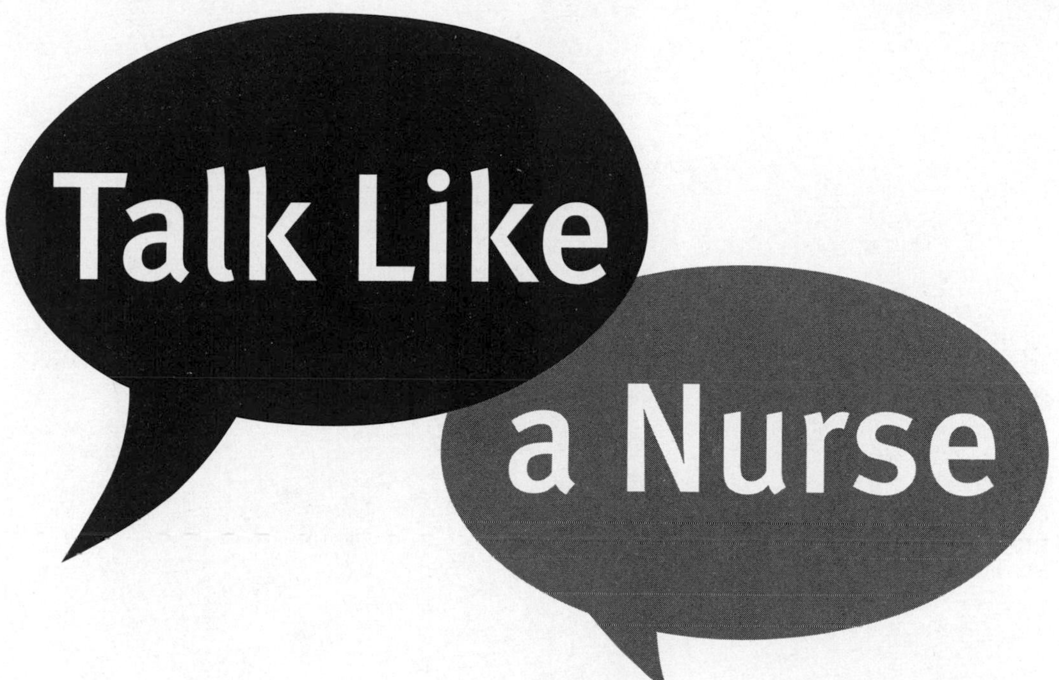

Talk Like a Nurse

Communication Skills Workbook

Susan Dandridge Bosher, PhD

Published by Kaplan Publishing, a division of Kaplan, Inc.
395 Hudson Street
New York, NY 10014

Printed in the United States of America
10 9 8 7 6 5 4 3 2 1
ISBN-13: 978-1-61865-450-2

Kaplan Publishing books are available at special quantity discounts to use for sales promotions, employee premiums, or educational purposes. For more information or to order books, please call the Simon & Schuster special sales department at 866-506-1949.

Contents

CHAPTER FOUR: Addressing Personal Health–Related Issues

Acknowledgments

This book would not have been possible without the nursing content and cultural insights so generously provided by **Isabella (Bella) Muhia**, BS, RN. Bella's unwavering commitment to creating materials to facilitate the success of multicultural and multilingual students in nursing was essential to the completion of this project. She devoted countless hours in the evenings, on the weekends, and over the summer months to help bring this project to fruition.

I am also grateful for the support provided by the Assistant Mentorship Program (AMP) at St. Catherine University, in St. Paul, Minnesota, which provided funding for Bella's participation in the project; and to St. Catherine University for granting me a semester-long sabbatical to resurrect and reinvigorate this book project, which in fact, began many years ago.

I have benefited tremendously over the years from the knowledge, wisdom, and support of many nurse educators and administrators who shared the vision of creating a more culturally and linguistically diverse nursing profession, in particular **Alice Swan**, **Margaret McLaughlin**, and **Margaret Dexheimer Pharris** at St. Catherine University. I am also indebted to the following nurse educators for their review of content and for materials they provided for many of the expansion activities in this book, in particular **Pamela Hamre** (for medication orders, telephone reports, and telephone orders); **Jeannine Mueller-Harmon** and **Corjena Cheung** (for diagnostic labels and their etiologies, nursing goals, desired outcomes, and nursing interventions); **Susan Ellen Campbell** and **Kathy Bell** (for change-of-shift reports); **Virginia McCarty** (for medication orders); and **Susan Forneris** (for input regarding the use of SBAR for change-of-shift reports).

Finally, I am grateful for having worked with an editor at Kaplan Publishing, **Dorothy Cummings**, who not only shared my excitement and enthusiasm for this project, but also provided me with support and encouragement that kept me going.

Introduction

Congratulations! By using this workbook, you are taking the first step in preparing for the specific communication needs of nurses in the United States. If English is not your native language, or if you speak a variety of English that is different from North American English, then this workbook is especially for you. Whether you are a pre-nursing candidate for an associate- or baccalaureate-degree nursing program in the United States, a U.S. nursing student, or an internationally educated nurse preparing to enter the U.S. workforce, *Talk Like a Nurse* will help you strengthen the language skills you will need on the job and will familiarize you with the culture of nursing in the United States. This workbook assumes that you are proficient in at least an intermediate level of general academic English.

Talk Like a Nurse addresses the language needs that you will find in the health care setting and in the work you will do as a nurse: medical/nursing vocabulary and abbreviations; medication orders; nursing care plans, including nursing diagnoses, goals, desired outcomes, and nursing interventions; telephone reports and orders; progress notes; documentation skills; and communicating effectively with clients, such as making small talk, understanding client talk, and using therapeutic communication and interviewing skills. This workbook also introduces you to different cultural perspectives on topics that will be important for you to know as a nurse, such as managing pain and addressing personal health–related issues.

Content Structure

To maximize your learning, *Talk Like a Nurse* introduces language skills and cultural perspectives through nursing content. This approach lets you learn about language and culture in a way that is authentic, practical, and relevant to your future career. It also gives you a head start in learning or reviewing nursing content that will help you succeed in both your program and your future career as a nurse. The chapters in this book follow the same basic structure:

- Each chapter begins with a **client scenario**, which introduces you to a client with a particular diagnosis and medical history who has recently been admitted to the hospital. Based on the client scenario, you will have the opportunity to think critically and holistically about providing care for this client. You will also practice understanding medication orders, labs, tests, nursing actions, and nursing plans of care.
- The nurse then determines a **nursing diagnosis** for the client, followed by activities for you to develop your understanding of nursing interventions and desired outcomes, as well as practice using the language of nursing diagnoses, goals, desired outcomes, and nursing interventions.

- For each client, there is a **telephone report** from the nurse to the clinician about a change in the client's condition. The clinician then responds with a **telephone order** to the nurse outlining changes that the nurse should make in the client's care. These sections include activities to develop your understanding of the telephone order and the telephone report.
- At the end of the shift, the nurse writes a **progress report** about the care that was provided to the client during the shift. The progress report is followed by activities for you to practice documenting client care.
- Each chapter also includes a section on communicating effectively with clients, beginning with a **dialog between the nurse and client**. After the dialog, specific communication skills are introduced, followed by activities challenging you to analyze the communication skills used in the dialog and to practice using them yourself.
- Each chapter concludes with a section on **culture in nursing**, which explores cultural differences in some aspect of client care.

Whether you are a pre-nursing student, nursing student, or internationally educated nurse whose native language is not English, you may face challenges beyond those of your peers and colleagues. We want you to succeed in nursing, and we hope that this workbook will help prepare you for success. We also hope that as you develop your skills to help others through nursing, you will help create a U.S. nursing profession that is more culturally diverse—and thus more culturally competent.

We wish you all the best on your important journey ahead!

Susan Dandridge Bosher, PhD
Isabella Muhia, BS, RN
June 2014
St. Paul, Minnesota

About the Author

Susan Bosher, PhD, is professor and director of ESL at St. Catherine University in St. Paul, Minnesota, where she has taught English for Cross-Cultural Nursing to pre-nursing ESL students since 2000. The author of *English for Nursing, Academic Skills* and co-editor of *Transforming Nursing Education: The Culturally Inclusive Environment*, she has conducted research on linguistic bias in multiple-choice test items on nursing exams. She has presented frequently at conferences and workshops on various topics related to ESL and nursing.

About the Contributor

Isabella Muhia, BS, RN (Nursing and Public Health), is a candidate for MSN, Nurse Educator concentration, at St. Catherine University in St. Paul, Minnesota. She served as teaching assistant in English for Cross-Cultural Nursing, a course for pre-nursing ESL students (2011), and as adjunct instructor in pathophysiology (2012–2013), both at St. Catherine University.

Thinking Holistically about Clients

1

Learning Objectives

- Thinking holistically about clients
- Making small talk with clients
- Learning medical/nursing abbreviations related to medication orders: Dose of medication
- Identifying medication orders, labs, tests, and nursing actions
- Recognizing subjective vs. objective data in assessing clients
- Documenting client care: Understanding characteristics of effective documentation and using 24-hour clock and metric system
- Understanding and using therapeutic communication skills effectively: Empathy, attending to the client, "I" statements, reflection, verbal reassurance, nonverbal reassurance, caring touch, and silence
- Recognizing cultural differences in therapeutic communication skills

Scenario #1

Client: African-American female, 35 yo

Diagnosis: Infection secondary to appendectomy

History: Hypertension, diabetes mellitus type 2, right toe ulcer

Mrs. Nina Jackson is a 35-year-old African-American female who was admitted to the **medical/surgical** unit with a **diagnosis** of **infection** secondary to **appendectomy**. The client had an appendectomy 1 week ago. The **admitting nurse** noted that the area around the **abdominal incision** is warm to touch and slightly red. Pt rated pain at 5 on a scale of 0 to 10. Pt has a history of HTN (**hypertension**) and DM (**diabetes mellitus**) **type 2.** She takes **insulin** to keep her BG (**blood glucose**) level **stable** and **adheres** to a diabetic diet. She has an Ⓡ (right) toe **ulcer** that has not healed for 6 weeks. The admitting nurse noted that her Ⓡ toe is swollen and contains **purulent exudate**^. Pt stated upon admission, "I feel weak in my knees and this toe ulcer is driving me crazy. I can barely feel my foot now and sometimes the pain is unbearable!" Pt rated toe pain at 10 on a scale of 0 to 10. She is **Full Code**. She is **allergic** to **sulfa** and eggs. She is scheduled for a chest x-ray because of recent **positive** (+) **Mantoux**. The **clinician** ordered these medications for her: 0.9% NS (**normal saline**)* IV running at 125 mL/hr to maintain **hydration** and **fluid balance**, enalapril 5 mg PO BID to **stabilize** high blood pressure, Extra Strength Tylenol† 500 mg PO PRN q4–6 hr to relieve pain, 1 multivitamin tablet PO daily to supplement vitamin and mineral intake, NPH insulin subcut per **insulin protocol** to **regulate** blood sugar, and cefazolin 2 g in D_5W 50 mL IVPB q8h to fight the infection. She needs to be scheduled for CBC lab. She also needs to have a blood glucose capillary sample TID AC. Her VS (**vital signs**) and O_2 sats should be checked q4h and she should be weighed daily. The abdominal incision **site** and toe ulcer, along with pain level, should be assessed. **Contact precautions** should be taken. She has **bathroom privileges** with **assist of 1**. A **wound consult** has been ordered for both the incision site and the toe ulcer. She also needs a **focused respiratory assessment** because of the (+) Mantoux. Mrs. Jackson is married and has two sons, 7 and 11 years old. She is a pleasant woman. She works as an accountant and loves playing video games with her sons. She is Baptist and active in her church.

^Purulent exudate, sometimes called pus, is a fluid composed of blood products and fragments of bacteria and dead tissue, formed by the body in reaction to infection.

*Normal saline is a 0.9% sterile solution of sodium chloride.

†Acetaminophen is the generic name for this medication. However, for extra strength, the brand name Tylenol is used.

Critical Thinking Skills: Thinking Holistically about Clients

Critical thinking and *critical judgment* in nursing refer to the cognitive skills necessary for problem-solving and decision-making in the clinical context. The nurse does the following:

- Gathers information about a client
- Assesses the information
- Draws tentative conclusions about the client's health issue
- Then generates and evaluates possible responses to the issue

Critical thinking requires that the nurse's assessment take into consideration individual differences to determine how to provide the most effective care for the client. Clinical judgment is the result of critical thinking.

Holistic nursing considers the client as a whole person. In other words, holistic nursing considers all the dimensions of the individual, including not only the person's physiological needs but also his or her psychosocial, spiritual, and cultural needs. The nurse uses information about the person's needs to provide holistic care that addresses all dimensions of the individual. The goal is to heal the whole person; therefore, to think holistically about an individual is part of thinking critically about the person's care.

▶ Activity 1.1: Thinking Holistically about Clients

Determine your answers to the following questions based on Scenario #1 about Mrs. Jackson. How would you incorporate an understanding of psychosocial information in your holistic care of the client?

1. From a physiological perspective, what is Mrs. Jackson likely to be most concerned about with regard to her illness?

   ____

   ____

2. From a psychosocial perspective, what is Mrs. Jackson likely to be most concerned about with regard to her illness?

   ____

   ____

3. What actions could the nurse plan to take to respond to Mrs. Jackson's psychosocial needs?

   ____

   ____

Using Language Effectively in Health Care Settings

For nurses to establish a positive relationship with a client, it is helpful to be able to make small talk.

Nurse Talk: Making Small Talk

Small talk, or social conversation, usually starts with neutral topics but, depending on the client and the situation, small talk could lead to more personal talk. Small talk helps to establish common ground between the nurse and client. It also helps to relax the client and foster a connection and level of comfort with the nurse. Clients are more likely to be responsive to a nurse with whom they feel comfortable.

▶ Activity 1.2: Making Small Talk—Identifying Topics for Small Talk

Determine your answers to the following questions.

1. Identify at least 3 neutral topics that you could discuss with Mrs. Jackson.

____

____

2. Write a comment or question that relates to each topic that you could discuss with Mrs. Jackson.

____

____

3. Based on the information in Scenario #1, identify 3–4 topics that you could discuss with Mrs. Jackson. Write a question that relates to each topic.

____

____

4. Write a comment about yourself that relates to each topic identified in #3 or ask a follow-up question of the client.

____

____

5. In addition to the information provided in Scenario #1, what are other sources of information about a client that could suggest possible topics for conversation?

____

____

6. When is it not appropriate to make "small talk" or to ask personal questions of clients?

____

____

Medical/Nursing Vocabulary

How many of the bolded medical/nursing words used in Scenario #1 about Mrs. Jackson do you already know? For those words you do not know, look them up in a nursing textbook, an English-language medical dictionary, or online resources. Refer to the definitions in the Answer Key for Chapter One, as needed.

Medical/Nursing Abbreviations

Identify as many of the abbreviations as you can from Scenario #1, about Mrs. Jackson. Refer, as needed, to the list of Medical/Nursing Abbreviations in the Appendix.

Expansion of Medical/Nursing Abbreviations: Medication Orders (Dose of Medication)

The medications that Mrs. Jackson is currently taking are included in Scenario #1. Abbreviations and acronyms are commonly used in medication orders.

Medication Orders

There are 7 parts to a medication order:

1. Full name of client
2. Date and time the medication order is written
3. Name of medication to be given
4. Dose of medication (how much medication is given)
5. Route of administration (how the medication is given)
6. Frequency of administration (when and how often the medication is given)
7. Signature of person writing the order

Note: *Dose* refers to the quantity of medication given to a client at a single time. *Dosage* refers to the amount or strength of the medication.

▶ Activity 1.3: Dose of Medication

Write the correct abbreviation in the blank for each word or phrase used in medication orders.

The first one has been done for you.

D_5W g gtt mcg mEq mg mL

1. mg milligram
2. ________ milliliter
3. ________ milliequivalent
4. ________ 5% dextrose in water
5. ________ gram
6. ________ microgram
7. ________ drop

Expansion of Scenario #1: Understanding Medication Orders, Labs, Tests, and Nursing Actions

When Mrs. Jackson is admitted to the hospital, she is assessed by the attending physician, who orders medications, labs (laboratory tests), and other tests for her. In addition, both the physician and the nurse who is assigned to care for Mrs. Jackson on the medical-surgical unit determine appropriate nursing actions. Some of these nursing actions are carried out by the nurse; some are carried out by the licensed practical or vocational nurse (LPN/LVN) or nursing assistive personnel (NAP); and some are carried out by other health care professionals.

▶ Activity 1.4: Identifying Medication Orders, Labs, Tests, and Nursing Actions in Scenario #1

Write down the medications that are ordered for Mrs. Jackson. Why is each medication ordered? What information is provided for each medication, and in what order? For each medication, write the information that is provided.

Medications

____

____

____

____

____

Write down the labs and other tests that have been ordered and the nursing actions that have been planned for Mrs. Jackson.

Labs/Tests

____

____

____

____

____

Nursing Actions

____

____

____

____

____

Expansion of Scenario #1: Plan of Care

When nursing students prepare for clinical practice, they often use forms like the Plan of Care shown in Figure 1-1 to record essential information about the client from the client's record and to plan the client's care. Note that the route of medication is not always specified on the Plan of Care because nurses would always refer to the medication administration record (MAR) before administering medications. This Plan of Care reflects care for Mrs. Jackson during the day shift on her first day at the hospital. The vital signs recorded were taken at the beginning of the shift.

Figure 1-1: Plan of Care
Scenario #1

ROOM	DIET	OTHER	T	P	RR	BP
2307	*Diabetic*	*Full Code* *Contact precautions* *Tylenol 500 mg PRN* *NPH insulin*	*98.8*	*87*	*16*	*130/90*

INITIALS	ACTIVITY	O_2 sats / NOTES
NJ	*Bathroom privileges with assist of 1*	

Dx*	IVs
Infection secondary to appendectomy	*0.9% NS at 125 mL/hr* *Cefazolin 2 g in D_5W* *50 mL PB q8h*

MHx†	LABS/TESTS/APPTS	ASSESSMENTS
Hypertension *DM II* *Ⓡ toe ulcer*	*Chest x-ray* *CBC* *BG capillary sample TID AC* *Wound consult*	*VS q4h* *Daily weight* *Abd incision site* *Toe ulcer* *Pain* *Focused respiratory*

MDs	TREATMENTS
Dr. Warren	*Wound care*

ALLERGY	PAIN	OUTPUTS
Sulfa *Eggs*	*5/10 (incision site)* *10/10 (toe)*	*N/A*

0700/1900	0800/2000	0900/2100	1000/2200	1100/1300	1200/2400
1 multivitamin	*Enalapril 5 mg*				
1300/0100	**1400/0200**	**1500/0300**	**1600/0400**	**1700/0500**	**1800/0600**

*Dx = diagnosis

†MHx = medical history

▶ Activity 1.5: Plan of Care: Planning for Client's Care

Answer the following questions with information that is provided in the Plan of Care regarding Mrs. Jackson.

1. What is Mrs. Jackson's diagnosis?

___

___

2. What is Mrs. Jackson's medical history?

___

___

3. How often and when is Mrs. Jackson given 5 mg of enalapril? How many hours apart are the 2 doses given? How many doses are given during the day shift? During the evening shift?

___

___

4. What medications does Mrs. Jackson receive intravenously?

___

___

5. What assessments are planned for Mrs. Jackson?

___

___

Nursing Diagnosis: Thinking Holistically about Mrs. Jackson

Based on the information provided in the client's record and the nurse's assessment* of the client, the nurse writes a nursing diagnosis and a goal for treating the client. The nurse also identifies nursing interventions and desired outcomes to accomplish that goal. In planning holistic care for Mrs. Jackson, the nurse identifies interventions that address Mrs. Jackson's psychosocial needs, as well as her physiologic needs. Review the list of interventions in Activity 1.6. Which nursing intervention reflects care of Mrs. Jackson's psychosocial needs?

*A physical assessment usually is conducted when a client is first admitted to the hospital, either a head-to-toe assessment or a focused assessment on a specific problem area, followed by a head-to-toe assessment, as needed. Information from this assessment is included in the client's record and is reviewed by the nurse caring for Mrs. Jackson.

Nursing Diagnosis: Impaired skin integrity related to inflammation and impaired circulation secondary to diabetes mellitus as manifested by the following: redness and swelling around suture line, purulent exudate on right toe ulcer, and client's complaints of intense toe pain.

Goal: Client will have improved skin integrity.

▶ Activity 1.6: Nursing Diagnosis: Nursing Interventions and Desired Outcomes

Match each Desired Outcome for Mrs. Jackson with the corresponding Nursing Intervention.

Write the letter of the Desired Outcome in the correct blank.

Nursing Intervention	Desired Outcome
1. __________ Nurse will offer client a back rub and teach client relaxation techniques by the end of shift.	a. Client will report decreased pain level of 2 (scale 0–10) in abdomen within 1 hour of analgesic administration.
2. __________ Nurse will teach client splinting* techniques by the end of shift.	b. Client will report decreased pain level of 2 (scale 0–10) in toe ulcer within 1 hour of analgesic administration.
3. __________ Nurse will administer pain medication and a cool pack to relieve abdominal pain during shift.	c. Client will report less anxiety by the end of shift.
4. __________ Nurse will clean toe ulcer, apply dressing, and elevate the foot during shift.	d. Client will demonstrate how to splint the abdominal wound by the end of shift.

*splinting = techniques to support a wound or sensitive area, especially during movement

Nursing Process and Nursing Care Plans: Subjective vs. Objective Data

Nursing Process

The nursing process is a systematic procedure used to provide nursing care. It consists of 5 components:

1. Assessment
2. Diagnosing
3. Planning
4. Implementation
5. Evaluation

In **assessment**, the nurse collects data about the client; in **diagnosing**, the nurse analyzes the data and determines a nursing diagnosis, using a set of diagnoses established by the North American Nursing Diagnosis Association (NANDA); in **planning**, the nurse creates a nursing care plan, which includes nursing interventions and desired outcomes for the client; in **implementation**, the nurse puts into action the interventions that have been identified in the care plan; in **evaluation**, the nurse evaluates the client's progress toward achieving the desired outcomes and thereby evaluates the effectiveness of the nursing care plan. More than one component can be involved at any given time in the nursing process (Figure 1-2).

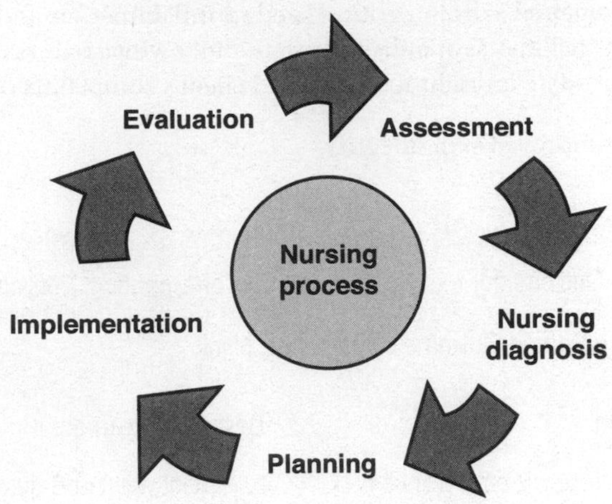

Figure 1-2: Nursing Process

Nursing Care Plans

Nursing care plans reflect the nursing process. They organize information about client care and specify the actions nurses take in providing care for the client. They also allow for continuity of care from one nurse to another. Care plans typically consist of 4 categories of information:

1. Nursing diagnoses
2. Goals/desired outcomes
3. Nursing interventions
4. Evaluation

Nursing care plans require a specialized kind of writing.

Student care plans tend to be longer and more detailed than care plans used by practicing nurses. Student care plans may include assessment data, rationales for nursing interventions, and supporting literature for each rationale.

Subjective vs. Objective Data

Gathering assessment data is the first step in preparing a nursing care plan. Assessment data is divided into 2 types: subjective data and objective data.

Subjective data refers to how the client experiences an illness or health problem. It includes feelings, values, beliefs, attitudes, and perceptions, as well as sensations that are apparent only to the person affected and can be described or verified only by that person. Subjective data are also referred to as **symptoms**. Some examples are feelings of inadequacy, concern about the illness, itching, and pain.

Objective data can be seen, heard, felt, or smelled by someone other than the person affected. They can be measured using some kind of standard—for example, blood pressure reading or observation of a skin lesion. Objective data are gathered during the health assessment to validate subjective data. They are also referred to as **signs**.

Information provided by other people, such as family members or other health care providers, can be either subjective or objective, depending on whether it is based on fact. For example, "Dad is very confused today" is subjective. However, "Dad couldn't remember his address or phone number today" is objective.

Note the subjective and objective ways of describing the same problem:

Subjective Data	Objective Data
"When I push myself to move, I feel weak all over."	Blood pressure 85/57 mm Hg Pulse 91 bpm Cool, clammy skin
"I feel like my stomach is being twisted and it's so painful."	Blood-tinged diarrhea Hyperactive bowel sounds in all 4 quadrants Vomited 70 mL yellow-tinged fluid
"It's hard for me to breathe."	Crackles heard over lung fields bilaterally Diminished lung sounds in middle and lower lobes bilaterally
Nephew stated: "He seems to be in some pain this evening."	Client grimaced and raised eyebrows during assessment.
"I would like to have Holy Communion with the priest."	Has a rosary around neck Holding hymn book

▶ Activity 1.7: Subjective vs. Objective Data

Read the statements listed here. Label each statement as subjective (**SUBJ**) or objective (**OBJ**).

1. __________ Mr. F has not had a bowel movement in 3 days.
2. __________ Mr. F complains of being constipated.
3. __________ Ms. G says she has a pain that comes and goes in her left eye.
4. __________ Both eyelids appear swollen.
5. __________ The wrist looks red.
6. __________ Mr. K says that the wrist does not hurt when he moves it.
7. __________ "I forget to take my pills."
8. __________ "I can't live without sugar in my food."
9. __________ Weight is 98 kg (215 lbs); gain of 4.5 kg (10 lbs).
10. __________ Blood pressure 190/100 mm Hg.

▶ Activity 1.8: Identifying Subjective and Objective Data

Review Scenario #1. Make 2 lists of assessment data regarding Mrs. Jackson: 1 list for subjective data and 1 list for objective data.

Subjective Data

____

____

____

Objective Data

____

____

____

Telephone Report

Nurses sometimes contact the clinician about a client by telephone—for example, when there is a medical emergency or when there is a significant or noteworthy change in the client's condition.

The nurse caring for Mrs. Jackson contacts the attending physician about a change in Mrs. Jackson's condition. Here is what the nurse reports to the physician, referred to as a *telephone report*:

> *Hello, Dr. Warren. This is Cheryl Soko, the nurse caring for Mrs. Nina Jackson, a 35-year-old woman, in Room 2307. She came in with an infection at her abdominal incision site following an appendectomy. She has a history of hypertension and diabetes mellitus type 2 and has a right toe ulcer. She is on enalapril PO, NPH insulin, 0.9% normal saline IV, and cefazolin IV piggyback. Her vital signs are stable except her temp, which is 101. She attempted turning herself in bed and started coughing but did not splint. As a result, some of her stitches opened up and there is some dehiscence* at the suture line. I suspect that the infection might get worse. How would you like to proceed with this situation?*

*dehiscence = the opening up of a surgical wound

Documentation of Telephone Report

After completing the telephone report, the nurse documents the date, the time, the person called, the person who received the information, what information was given, and what information was received. Figure 1-3 shows the documentation of the telephone report about Mrs. Jackson.

Figure 1-3: Documentation of Telephone Report

07-04-13 0810 Nina Jackson. VSS except T 101. Dehiscence at suture line after turning in bed and coughing. Infection at abdominal incision. Dr. Warren notified via phone.---C. Soko, RN

Telephone Order

In response to telephone reports, clinicians usually change medication and other orders for the client. Here is the attending physician's response to the nurse's report about Mrs. Jackson, referred to as a *telephone order* (T.O.). Note that spoken delivery of medication orders differs in some ways from written orders.

> *Hello, Cheryl. From your brief summary on Mrs. Jackson in Room 2307, discontinue the cefazolin IV and start infusing* immediately 1,000 milligrams of vancomycin IV piggyback every 12 hours. I will send the resident physician to inspect the abdominal wound. She will apply adhesive on the edges and cover it with abdominal dressing. Put the client on bed rest. Monitor her vitals every 30 minutes and give her 400 milligrams of ibuprofen by mouth immediately. I will have the resident physician also check on the ulcer. Thank you.*
>
> *infusing = injecting a solution for therapeutic purposes through a person's vein

Documentation of Telephone Order

The nurse must document telephone orders from the clinician. Figure 1-4 shows the nurse's documentation of the telephone order about Mrs. Jackson, referred to as a *telephone order report.*

Figure 1-4: Telephone Order Report

1. D/C cefazolin IV
2. Start vancomycin 1,000 mg IVPB q12hr stat
3. Administer ibuprofen 400 mg PO stat
4. Put pt on bed rest
5. Monitor VS q30 min

07-04-13 0825

T.O. from Dr. Warren/Cheryl Soko, RN

▶ Activity 1.9: Understanding Telephone Order Report

Answer the following questions based on the telephone order report about Mrs. Jackson.

1. Which medication is discontinued for Mrs. Jackson?

   ____

2. What new medications are ordered for Mrs. Jackson?

   ____

3. When is Mrs. Jackson given the new medications?

   ____

   ____

4. How often are Mrs. Jackson's vitals taken? In Scenario #1, how often were vitals taken? Why is there a difference in frequency, do you think?

   ____

   ____

5. How much ibuprofen is Mrs. Jackson given? In Scenario #1, how much Extra Strength Tylenol was Mrs. Jackson given? Why is there a difference in pain medication, do you think?

   ____

   ____

6. Why do you think Mrs. Jackson is put on bed rest?

   ____

   ____

Documentation of Client Care: Progress Note

At the end of the shift, the nurse documents the care that was given to the client in the form of a progress note. Here is the progress note about the care that was provided to Mrs. Jackson.

Progress Note

Identify Problem(s)

Pain from dehiscence of abdominal wound, risk for infection secondary to dehiscence, right toe ulcer, and anxiety secondary to dehiscence

Desired Outcome(s)

Pt will report decreased pain level of 2 (scale 0–10) in abdomen and toe ulcer within 1 hour of analgesic administration.

Pt's blood glucose will be controlled using insulin during shift.

O_2 saturation will improve to above 90% by the end of shift.

Pt will remain free from falls or injury throughout shift.

Pt will report less anxiety by the end of shift.

Evaluation

VSS. Surgical site pain secondary to dehiscence rated at 5 out of 10. Adhesive and abdominal dressing put on surgical site per MD's order and site was assessed by resident physician. Pt was anxious after dehiscence occurred. Pt was given ibuprofen 400 mg PO at 0845 per MD's order. Toe ulcer has purulent exudate and serous* discharge. BG is 120 mg/dL. SSI administered today per protocol. Pt on diabetic diet but eats only 50% of meals. O_2 sats 95%. On bed rest. Pt denied† nausea and vomiting, and her bowel sounds are active.‡ Pain affecting her ability to sleep, but after ibuprofen she had a 2 hr nap. Pt encouraged to take fluids and is being turned q2h. Her family is supportive,§ and attending physician updated her husband on progress.

Plan

Continue to monitor client health status and progress. Continue to administer medications per MAR. Reinforce teaching pt about wound care and splinting and relaxation techniques. Provide quiet, healing environment for pt, maintain on bed rest to promote well-being, continue to turn q2h, and encourage fluids. Provide opportunities for client to spend time with her children. Discuss plan of care with pt and husband. Encourage pt to inform nurse of any concerns regarding her health and care.

*serous = bodily fluid that is thin and watery, pale yellow, and transparent

^SSI = sliding-scale insulin

†denied = When a client denies a symptom, it means the client reports that he or she is not experiencing it.

‡active = irregular gurgling noises in the abdomen occurring about every 5 to 20 seconds, indicating bowels are within normal limits

§supportive = provides emotional assistance or any other assistance that will aid in promotion of health

▶ **Activity 1.10: Providing Holistic Care**

Determine your answers to the following questions based on the care provided to Mrs. Jackson.

How does the plan (of care) in the progress note reflect holistic care of Mrs. Jackson? How have Mrs. Jackson's psychosocial and physiological needs been addressed in the plan?

____

____

____

____

____

Expansion of Documentation of Client Care: Characteristics of Effective Documentation

The client record is a legal document that can be used in court as evidence. Therefore, nurses must meet certain legal standards when they record information about client care. Document as often as required by the health care agency where you work and as soon as possible after completing an assessment or intervention. Never document before providing nursing care. Documentation should be factual, accurate, complete, current, and organized. Documentation must identify that the client received individualized, goal-directed nursing care based on nursing assessment. Record only information that is relevant to the client's current health problems and care. Do not record personal information that has no effect on the client's current condition, as that could be considered an invasion of the client's privacy and cause for a lawsuit.

Hospitals and other health care facilities now use electronic medical records (EMRs), which are characterized by computerized charting with pull-down menus and boxes to be checked or filled out in order to record assessment data and document standard care. Normal responses for various assessments and options for standard care are included in the computer program. Despite the widespread use of computerized charting, some aspects of client care, such as progress notes, are still typed into the electronic record. Progress notes are used to document abnormal findings, also referred to as *charting by exception* (CBE). In addition, some facilities have not transitioned from paper records, especially home health care agencies.

Documentation by Hand

In facilities where documentation is done by hand, make sure that your entries are easy to read. Handwriting that is not legible can be misread by other health care professionals, which can result in misinterpretation of essential information. Use black ink in case photocopies need to be made and so that any changes are easy to identify. If you make a mistake in your recording, do not erase or use correction fluid. Draw 1 line through the mistake and write the words *mistaken entry* next to it, followed by your initials or name. Do not write the word *error* when indicating a recording mistake because the word *error* could imply that a clinical error was made. Write on every line, but do not write between lines. If there is any blank space left over on a line, draw a line through it, so that no one can add or change any information at another time. Sign each recording with your name and title. For nursing students, the abbreviation NS is used; for registered nurses, the abbreviation RN is used. (In computerized charting, the computer adds your name, your title, the date, and the time.) Finally, correct spelling is essential for accuracy.

For example, *Librium* and *lithium* and *Celexa* and *Celebrex* are similar in spelling, but refer to different medications. In addition, incorrect spelling can give a negative impression to colleagues and decrease the nurse's credibility. Look up any words you are unsure about in a dictionary. (Although computerized charting has a spell check function, it will not catch incorrect words that are spelled correctly.)

Date and Time

The date and time of each recording should be documented. Use the 24-hour clock, also known as military time, to avoid any confusion about whether a time was a.m. or p.m. For example, in the conventional way of writing time in the United States, 9:00 could refer to 9:00 a.m. or 9:00 p.m. In the 24-hour system, there is no potential for confusion between morning and afternoon hours.

In the 24-hour system, morning times do not change, but 0 is written before the first number, up through the number 9. Colons are not used to separate minutes from the hour. For example, 9:00 a.m. = 0900 (pronounced oh-nine-hundred) and 11:30 a.m. = 1130. Afternoon and evening times are calculated differently. Except for the noon and midnight hours, simply add 12 to the hour. For example, 1:30 p.m. = 1330 and 10:30 p.m. = 2230. Midnight is written as 2400. Noon is written as 1200.

▶ Activity 1.11: Understanding the 24-Hour Clock

Convert the following times from the 12-hour clock to the 24-hour clock. The first one has been done for you.

12-Hour Clock	24-Hour Clock
1. 4:40 a.m.	1. 0440
2. 4:40 p.m.	2. ________
3. 10:10 a.m.	3. ________
4. 10:10 p.m.	4. ________
5. 12:30 a.m.	5. ________
6. 12:30 p.m.	6. ________

Metric System

In nursing, the metric system is used. It consists of the following basic units of measurement—the *meter* (for length), the *liter* (for volume), and the *gram* (for weight)—and is based on units of 10. Each unit of measurement can be multiplied by 10 or divided by 10 to form other units. Latin prefixes are used to designate subdivisions of the basic unit. For example, *deci* refers to 1/10; *centi* to 1/100; and *milli* to 1/1,000. Greek prefixes are used to designate multiples of the basic unit. For example, *deka* refers to 10; *hecto* to 10, and *kilo* to 1,000.

To convert measurements to the metric system from other systems used in the United States, such as the apothecary system and common household measurements, refer to this chart.

Household/Apothecary	Metric
1 tablespoon	15 mL (milliliters)
1 fluid ounce	30 mL
1 pint	500 mL
1 quart	1,000 mL
1 gallon	4,000 mL
1 ounce	30 g (grams)
1.1 pound (lb)	500 g
2.2 lbs	1,000 g (1 kg or kilogram)
1 inch	2.5 cm (centimeter)

▶ Activity 1.12: Understanding the Metric System

Match the metric measurement with the corresponding household measurement. Write the letter of the metric measurement in the correct blank. The first one has been done for you.

Household Measurement	Metric Measurement
1. ___c___ half a cup	a. 5 cm
2. ______ 2 inches	b. 90 g
3. ______ 4 inches	c. 125 mL
4. ______ 11 pounds	d. 1,500 mL
5. ______ 2 fluid ounces	e. 30 mL
6. ______ 2 tablespoons	f. 60 mL
7. ______ 3 ounces	g. 10 cm
8. ______ 3 pints	h. 5 kg

Communication Skills: Therapeutic Communication

Communicating with clients is an essential part of nursing. Read the dialog between the nurse and Mrs. Jackson, which takes place during the shift. The nurse uses various therapeutic communication skills to help Mrs. Jackson cope with her situation.

Dialog between Nurse and Mrs. Jackson

Nurse: *(enters the room) Good morning, Mrs. Jackson. (smiles)*

Mrs. Jackson: *Hello… (frowns and looks away)*

Nurse: *I see that you seem upset. (sits down, moves chair close to Mrs. Jackson, establishes eye contact with client, and leans in) Could you please tell me what is going on?*

Mrs. Jackson: *Well, my problems are getting to be too much…*

Nurse: *You're concerned about your health? (Nurse maintains eye contact.)*

Mrs. Jackson: *Yes, I've had this toe ulcer for a long time. I accidentally bumped my toe and now the sore won't go away! To make matters worse, this abdominal wound started opening up and I saw some of my intestines! Don't those surgeons know what they are doing? (raises her voice and points at her abdominal wound)*

Nurse: *When did you bump your toe?*

Mrs. Jackson: *I bumped it 6 weeks ago.*

Nurse: *Did you do anything to make it feel better?*

Mrs. Jackson: *I put some salt* and a bandage on it, but the pain hasn't gone away. It's gotten worse.*

Nurse: *Your toe is still in pain? (Nurse squats to visually inspect the toe.) I will take a closer look shortly. The abdominal wound opened up because, while you were turning, a lot of pressure was put on the stitches and they could no longer hold together. The dressing will help keep everything in place until the resident can look at it and tell us what to do. How is your pain now?*

Mrs. Jackson: *It seems like the ibuprofen helped; it's not hurting as much.*

Nurse: *How would you rate your pain on a scale of 0 to 10?*

Mrs. Jackson: *About a 5. But, now that the wound on my tummy† has opened up, I don't know if I will be able to care for my toe. My blood sugar has also been on a roller coaster. I'm completely worn out with all these health problems. (teary-eyed)*

Nurse: *(places her hand on Mrs. Jackson's shoulder and uses a quiet tone of voice) I understand that it has been quite challenging for you with all that you have been going through, and indeed health concerns can be very draining. I just want to let you know that you are in the right place because my team and I will do our very best to care for you. (silent moment)*

Mrs. Jackson: *I appreciate it. Just go nice and easy with me.*

Nurse: *Yes, Mrs. Jackson. Please let me know if you have any questions or concerns. Now you can get ready for your family's visit. They are coming soon.*

*Salt is an alternative type of antiseptic; it is sometimes used as a home remedy, especially for skin injuries—in this case a skin ulcer. Mrs. Jackson's use of salt illustrates that people try interventions at home to feel better before seeking medical treatment when issues have escalated.

†tummy = abdomen

▶ Activity 1.13: Analyzing Effectiveness of Communication

Determine your answers to the following questions about the effectiveness of the nurse's communication with Mrs. Jackson in the dialog.

1. What is Mrs. Jackson concerned about?

____

____

2. How does the nurse encourage Mrs. Jackson to speak about her concerns?

____

____

3. Is the nurse able to address Mrs. Jackson's concerns? Why or why not?

____

____

4. Do you have any suggestions for how the nurse could be more effective in her communication with Mrs. Jackson? If so, explain.

____

____

Expansion of Dialog (Therapeutic Communication Skills): Empathy, Attending to the Client, "I" Statements, Reflection, Verbal Reassurance, Nonverbal Reassurance, Caring Touch, and Silence

Therapeutic communication is used by nurses to help clients cope with their situation as well as recover their independence. Some therapeutic communication skills help to build the client's trust in the nurse; other skills encourage clients to talk about their feelings and concerns; other skills help clients establish personal goals and realize them.

Empathy

Empathy is the ability to experience a situation through the eyes and feelings of another person. Empathy allows the nurse to understand the client more deeply, including the client's psychosocial and physiological needs; it also allows the client to feel greater acceptance. The nurse's ability to respond empathetically to a client is an essential part of therapeutic communication.

Attending to the Client

The first step in therapeutic communication is attending to the client or creating a comfortable and supportive environment, free from all distractions. Such an environment allows the nurse to give all of his or her attention to the client.

Some ways to create a supportive environment include finding a place to talk that is private; making sure your client is physically comfortable (e.g., in a chair or in bed); putting yourself at the same eye level as your client (e.g., sit in a chair rather than stand); sitting close enough to easily hear your client and vice versa; reducing or eliminating outside distractions (e.g., close the door, ask to turn off the TV); and avoiding looking at records, charts, and questions written on paper, which may distract you from your client or make your client feel that you are not listening.

▶ Activity 1.14: Analyzing Dialog for Empathy and Attending Behaviors

Determine your answers to the following questions about the nurse's use of empathy and attending behaviors.

1. In what specific ways does the nurse encourage Mrs. Jackson to talk about her feelings and concerns?

   ____

   ____

2. Does the nurse respond empathetically to the client? If so, how?

   ____

   ____

3. Does the nurse address both the client's physiological and psychosocial needs? If so, how?

   ____

   ____

4. Do you think the nurse has gained the client's trust? If so, what evidence indicates that the client trusts the nurse?

   ____

   ____

5. How does the nurse attend to Mrs. Jackson in the dialog? What specific attending behaviors does the nurse use?

   ____

   ____

"I" Statements

"I" statements are statements that begin with the pronoun "I." These statements help nurses avoid judging a client or expressing disapproval, which are blocks to therapeutic communication. (See "Communication Skills: Blocks to Therapeutic Communication" in Chapter Two.) "I" statements allow nurses to own their own feelings and concerns; they are alternatives to "you" statements, or statements that begin with the pronoun "you," which often sound judgmental.

For example, a nurse notices that a client did not eat anything at mealtime. Compare the difference between a "you" statement and an "I" statement in response to that situation:

"You" Statement	**"I" Statement**
"You didn't eat anything for lunch. Why not?"	"I noticed you didn't eat anything for lunch. Is something wrong?"

▶ Activity 1.15: Analyzing "I" Statements

Which of the statements just listed is more effective and why? Look back at the Dialog between Nurse and Mrs. Jackson. Identify any examples of "I" (or "you") statements in the dialog. Are there other instances where the nurse could have used "I" statements?

____

____

____

____

____

Use of "I" Statements

There are certain situations in which "I" statements are particularly useful:

- Discussing feelings ("I hear you saying that . . .")
- Giving suggestions ("I think you could . . .")
- Asking the client to comply ("I would like you to . . .")
- Requesting information ("I would like to ask you some questions . . .")
- Giving your opinion ("I think that . . .")
- Expressing your feelings or concerns in an assertive way with colleagues and co-workers ("I feel that . . .")

"I" statements can be overdone. The nurse should not begin every observation with "I notice" or every expression of concern with "I feel," or the interaction with the client will sound formulaic and artificial. Be selective about when to use "I" statements.

Use of "We" Statements

The use of "we," and the related forms "us" and "our," does not promote therapeutic communication. Their use is considered patronizing, even condescending, toward the client, and blocks therapeutic communication. (See "Communication Skills: Blocks to Therapeutic Communication" in Chapter Two.)

Inappropriate	**Appropriate**
It's time for *our* bath.	It's time for *your* bath.

▶ Activity 1.16: Using "I" Statements

Practice using "I" statements. Transform the ineffective statements on the left into effective "I" statements. The first one has been done for you.

Ineffective Statement	Effective "I" Statement
1. "Mr. Nguyen, you should get ready for your bath now."	1. "Mr. Nguyen, I'd like you to get ready for your bath now."
2. "You frequently miss your appointments."	2. ______________________
3. "You haven't eaten anything on your plate."	3. ______________________
4. "You are not very clear."	4. ______________________
5. "Don't we look nice today."	5. ______________________
6. "It's time for us to get ready for your family's visit."	6. ______________________

Reflection

Reflection refers to statements in which the nurse reflects or gives back to the client feelings that the client has stated or implied in his or her previous message. Reflection allows the client to explore his or her own feelings. When the nurse restates the client's feelings or verbalizes what the client has implied, the client often responds by exploring his or her feelings more deeply.

Client's Statement: Example #1	Nurse's Response
It's been such a long day. I've been given so many tests and I still don't know the results. The doctor hasn't even come to see me. It's scary.	It's *scary* for you.

In this response, the nurse reflects back to the client feelings that the client actually stated ("scary").

Client's Statement: Example #2	Nurse's Response
It's been such a long day. I've been given so many tests and I still don't know the results. The doctor hasn't even come to see me.	You sound *concerned.*

In this response, the nurse verbalizes feelings that the client has implied. However, the nurse states those feelings in general, rather than specifically naming them. The nurse would *not* say, "You sound *scared,*" as the nurse should not guess what the client is feeling. By stating in general what the client has implied ("You sound *concerned*"), the nurse encourages the client to name his or her own feelings and to explore them more deeply.

Use of Verbs in Reflection

The verbs "be" and "feel" suggest certainty and should be used to respond to feelings that are *stated* by the client. The verbs "sound" and "seem" suggest possibility and should be used to respond to feelings that are *implied* by the client.

Client's Statement	Nurse's Response
Feelings are stated: "It's scary."	Use verbs *be, feel* (certainty): "It's scary for you."
Feelings are implied: "It's been such a long day."	Use verbs *sound, seem* (possibility): "You *sound* concerned."

In Example #1, in which the client states explicitly his or her feelings, the nurse would *not* say: "It *seems* scary for you." Such a response would suggest that the nurse was not listening to what the client said or that the nurse doubts how the client is feeling.

In Example #2, in which the client implies his or her feelings, the nurse would *not* say: "You *are* concerned." To do so would suggest that the nurse knows exactly how the client is feeling.

Use of "You" Statements in Reflection

Reflecting statements sometimes begin with "you," in contrast to "I" statements, in which the nurse avoids the use of "you." To avoid confusing when to use "I" statements and when to use "you" statements, consider the purpose or function of the 2 skills—that is, what you (the nurse) are trying to communicate to the client. Nurses use "I" statements to own their *own* feelings and concerns and to avoid judging or blaming the client. Nurses use "you" statements in reflection to help *clients* explore their own feelings. If you get confused about which pronoun to use for what skill, think first about the purpose of the interaction—that is, what you (the nurse) are trying to communicate to the client.

As with "I" statements, nurses need to be selective about when to use reflection or they could risk sounding like a parrot, repeating any and all feeling words a client says. If a nurse overuses reflection, the client will quickly realize that the nurse is not being genuine. The nurse must listen carefully to the client and consider a variety of factors, such as the client's cultural background, age, and sex, when deciding when, what, and how to reflect.

▶ Activity 1.17: Analyzing Dialog for Reflection

Look back at the Dialog between Nurse and Mrs. Jackson. Identify any examples of reflection in the dialog. What is the effect of the reflection? Are there other instances where the nurse could have used reflection?

____

____

____

____

____

▶ Activity 1.18: Using Reflection

Practice using reflection in response to clients' statements. Respond to the client's statements on the left with reflections by the nurse. The first one has been done for you.

Client's Statement	Nurse's Reflection
1. "I don't want to talk about anything. Just go away."	1. "You don't want to talk?" (with rising intonation)
2. "I'm so angry with myself."	2. ______________________
3. "Why do you care? I'm just going to die."	3. ______________________
4. (*crying*) "I'll never get better."	4. ______________________
5. (*sadly*) "Nobody cares about me. No one visits me here."	5. ______________________
6. "Nurse, what time is it? The doctor was supposed to be here this morning."	6. ______________________

▶ Activity 1.19: Considering Use of Reflection

Determine your answers to the following questions.

1. Is it difficult for you to use reflection? Why or why not?

____

____

2. Are there some feelings that are harder to reflect? Or easier? If so, explain.

____

____

3. Is reflection easier to use in some nursing situations? More difficult? If so, explain.

____

____

4. Are there cultural reasons why a nurse might have difficulty talking about feelings? Are there cultural reasons why a client might have difficulty talking about feelings? If so, explain.

____

____

Verbal Reassurance

Verbal reassurance is used to communicate positive and truthful messages to the client, such as the nurse is listening, the client's concerns are real and important, the nurse understands the client's concerns, the client is being treated like a person, good care is being given, certain changes are normal (e.g., a slow recovery from a stroke), and there is hope.

Reassurance, however, must be real and truthful; otherwise, it becomes false reassurance, a block to therapeutic communication. (See "Communication Skills: Blocks to Therapeutic Communication" in Chapter Two.)

▶ Activity 1.20: Analyzing Dialog for Verbal Reassurance

Look back at the Dialog between Nurse and Mrs. Jackson. Identify any examples of verbal reassurance in the dialog. What is the effect of the verbal reassurance? Are there other instances where the nurse could have used verbal reassurance?

___

___

___

___

___

▶ Activity 1.21: Using Verbal Reassurance

Practice using verbal reassurance. For each of the client's statements on the left, provide reassurance by the nurse that is real and truthful to the client. The first one has been done for you.

Client's Statement	Nurse's Response
1. "My stroke was weeks ago, and I still haven't recovered. I don't think I'll ever get better."	1. "I know you are concerned, but it can take many months to recover from a stroke. You are making steady progress."
2. "Nobody here cares what happens to me."	2. ______________________
3. "I heard on the radio that there is a shortage of nurses at this hospital. What kind of care will I get here after surgery?"	3. ______________________
4. "What difference does it make? I'm just a number here anyway."	4. ______________________
5. "My foot is in a lot of pain; I can hardly walk. I'm worried that it will never get better."	5. ______________________
6. "My doctor gave me a prescription for pain medication, but I haven't taken any. I'm concerned I might get addicted."	6. ______________________

Nonverbal Reassurance

Nurses can also communicate reassurance nonverbally, through visual, auditory, and kinesthetic communication.

Visual types of nonverbal communication, or communication the client can see, include the following: maintaining an "open" body posture (not crossing arms and legs), leaning forward, nodding head in an affirmative way, smiling (at appropriate times), looking concerned, and maintaining eye contact.

Auditory forms of nonverbal communication, or communication the client can hear, include the following: vocalizing "um-hmm" while listening to the client and using a quiet tone of voice and/or a relaxed rate of speech.

Kinesthetic types of nonverbal communication, or communication the client can feel, often involve touch: shaking hands to say hello and touching the client's lower or upper arm, shoulder, or hand. Sometimes putting an arm around the client can be appropriate.

When nonverbal reassurance accompanies verbal reassurance, it should be consistent with the verbal message. For example, the nurse should maintain eye contact with the client to show she or he cares and is listening carefully, rather than look around the room. Nonverbal communication is reassuring only when it communicates the same positive and truthful message as verbal reassurance.

▶ Activity 1.22: Analyzing Dialog for Nonverbal Reassurance

Look back at the dialog between the nurse and Mrs. Jackson. Identify any examples of nonverbal reassurance in the dialog that are combined with verbal reassurance. Are there other instances of nonverbal reassurance? If so, what are they? What is the effect of the nonverbal reassurance? Are there other instances where the nurse could have used nonverbal reassurance?

____

____

____

____

____

▶ Activity 1.23: Using Nonverbal Reassurance

Redo the activity on using verbal reassurance (Activity 1.21). This time, in addition to providing verbal reassurance, provide nonverbal reassurance, as well. Write out a variety of visual, auditory, and kinesthetic ways of communicating reassurance. The first one has been done for you.

Client's Statement	Nurse's Response
1. "My stroke was weeks ago, and I still haven't recovered. I don't think I'll ever get better."	1. *(leaning forward; maintaining eye contact)* "I know you are concerned, but it can take many months to recover from a stroke. You are making steady progress."
2. "Nobody here cares what happens to me."	2. ______________________
3. "I heard on the radio that there is a shortage of nurses at this hospital. What kind of care will I get here after surgery?"	3. ______________________
4. "What difference does it make? I'm just a number here anyway."	4. ______________________
5. "My foot is in a lot of pain; I can hardly walk. I'm worried that it will never get better."	5. ______________________
6. "My doctor gave me a prescription for pain medication, but I haven't taken any. I'm concerned I might get addicted."	6. ______________________

Caring Touch

There are 2 kinds of touch in nursing: procedural and caring. **Procedural touch** is touching clients during regular nursing procedures, such as while giving an injection or while providing physical care such as turning the client over in bed. Unless there are certain cultural or religious restrictions around procedural touch, clients usually expect and accept to be touched by nurses for procedural purposes.

In contrast, **caring touch** is the use of touch for therapeutic purposes, to encourage the expression of feelings. Caring touch can be used to convey nonverbal reassurance or more broadly a message of concern. Caring touch helps to build trust in the nurse that is essential in therapeutic communication. However, caring touch can sometimes be misunderstood by clients.

▶ Activity 1.24: Analyzing Dialog for Caring Touch

Look back at the dialog between the nurse and Mrs. Jackson. Identify any examples of caring touch in the dialog. What is the effect of the caring touch? Are there other instances where caring touch would have been inappropriate?

____

____

____

____

____

Silence

Silence can be a very effective therapeutic communication skill when it is used appropriately by the nurse. It allows the client time to process information, gather his or her thoughts, or search for the right words.

Silence can be overused either by happening too often or by lasting too long. Usually, 5–10 seconds of silence is all the client needs before he or she takes a turn to speak. Silence is often combined with nonverbal reassurance by the nurse, such as nodding the head or placing a hand on the client's shoulder.

▶ Activity 1.25: Analyzing Dialog for Silence

Look back at the Dialog between Nurse and Mrs. Jackson. Identify any examples of silence in the dialog. What is the effect of the silence? Are there other instances in which silence would have been inappropriate?

____

____

____

____

____

Culture in Nursing: Cultural Differences in Therapeutic Communication (Nonverbal Communication, Use of Touch, and Silence)

There are many cultural differences in the use of therapeutic communication, in particular, nonverbal communication, touch, and silence.

Cultural Differences in Nonverbal Communication

With regard to nonverbal communication, some common gestures in mainstream U.S. culture are inappropriate in other cultures. For example, touching a child on the top of the head is taboo in cultures that believe spirits enter and leave the body through the head. The "A-okay" sign is obscene in some cultures.

Other examples of nonverbal behavior may have different meanings in different cultures. For example, smiling may not always communicate pleasure; in some cultures, people smile when they are embarrassed.

Eye contact is perhaps the most frequently cited cultural difference in nonverbal communication. In some cultures, eye contact with someone older or of a higher status is considered disrespectful. In mainstream U.S. culture, eye contact shows that you are listening.

Nurses need to be aware of cultural differences in nonverbal communication in order to understand their clients' use of nonverbal communication and how their clients might interpret their own use of nonverbal communication.

▶ Activity 1.26: Considering Cultural Differences in Nonverbal Communication

Determine your answers to the following questions.

1. Have you ever misunderstood someone from another culture because of his or her use of nonverbal communication? If so, describe what happened.

   ____

   ____

2. Have you ever been misunderstood by someone from another culture because of your use of nonverbal communication? If so, describe what happened.

   ____

   ____

3. Has your use of nonverbal communication changed over time? If so, in what ways and why?

   ____

   ____

4. Is it difficult for you to use any of the examples of nonverbal communication discussed in the Nonverbal Reassurance section in this chapter? If so, which ones and why?

   ____

   ____

Cultural Differences in the Use of Touch

Some students have difficulty with the use of touch. They may be from cultural or religious backgrounds that do not encourage physical touch, especially between members of opposite sexes. Or they may be from cultures that encourage more physical touch than is the norm in the United States. Regardless of culture, some students may be from families that do not use touch to show affection, or they may simply be shy and uncomfortable with touch. The use of touch is a skill that is developed with experience. Its effective use depends on how comfortable the nurse is in initiating the touch, as well as how comfortable the client is in receiving it.

▶ Activity 1.27: Considering Cultural Differences in the Use of Touch

Determine your answers to the following questions.

1. Is it difficult for you to use touch with clients? Why or why not?

____

____

2. Is procedural or caring touch more difficult for you? Why?

____

____

3. Are there some nursing situations or clients that make it easier for you to use touch? Or harder to use touch?

____

____

4. How could you use touch–both procedural and caring–with a client who seems uncomfortable with touch?

____

____

5. If you are uncomfortable with touch, how could you learn to use touch effectively, both procedural and caring?

____

____

Cultural Differences in the Use of Silence

There are also cultural differences in the use of silence. Silence is viewed in many cultures as a normal part of a conversation, even as a sign of respect, whereas in mainstream U.S. culture, many people are uncomfortable with silence. The style of conversation that is common in the United States is sometimes compared to a game of tennis because of the rapid, nonstop exchange of words between the speaker and listener. Someone from a culture with a slower pace of conversation, with a speed more like the sport of bowling, might wait for a pause or a brief moment of silence to enter the conversation.

▶ Activity 1.28: Considering Cultural Differences in the Use of Silence

Determine your answers to the following questions.

1. Have you ever misunderstood others because of the lack of silence in a conversation? If so, describe what happened.

___

___

2. Is the conversational style in your culture more like tennis or bowling? In what ways?

___

___

3. Have you ever been misunderstood by someone from another culture because of your use of silence? If so, describe what happened.

___

___

4. Has your use of silence changed over time? If so, in what ways and why?

___

___

Chapter One Answer Key

Activity 1.1: Thinking Holistically about Clients

1. Mrs. Jackson has several ailments that are occurring simultaneously (infection after an appendectomy and a right toe ulcer that is painful and won't go away) in addition to 2 serious illnesses (hypertension and diabetes mellitus type 2).

2. Mrs. Jackson might be most concerned about losing her job because she is back in the hospital. Also, she has some serious health challenges that will continue to cause her some anxiety when she returns home. She might be concerned about the effect her illness will have on her family, as she has 2 children (7 and 11 years old). Because Mrs. Jackson is on contact precautions, she might be concerned about how her children will perceive her as a caregiver. She might also be experiencing some anxiety due to having been dependent on others while she was recovering from surgery, feelings that will only increase now that she is back in the hospital.

3. Because Mrs. Jackson is active in her church, the nurse could ask Mrs. Jackson whether someone has contacted her church pastor to visit her. The nurse could also ask her about her support system at home, such as who is caring for her children while she is in the hospital.

Activity 1.2: Making Small Talk—Identifying Topics for Small Talk

1. A weather event; a recent civic event; a human interest story in the news

2. "Did you have any damage in the storm last week?" "Did you hear about the..." and "Isn't that an interesting story about..."

3. **Topics:** (1) Mrs. Jackson is married and has 2 sons, 7 and 11 years old. (2) She loves playing video games with her sons. (3) She works as an accountant. (4) She is Baptist and active in her church. **Questions:** (1) "Do you have any children, Mrs. Jackson?" (2) "How do you like to spend your time with them?" (3) "What work do you do?" (4) "Do you participate in a faith community?"

4. **Comments or Follow-up Questions:** (1) "I have 2 nephews about the same age." (2) "When they come over, they love to play with my cats." (3) "How long have you worked as an accountant?" (4) "How long have you been a member of this church?"

5. Photos, cards, flowers, and books in the room could also be topics of conversation, as in the following conversation starters: "What a handsome boy. Is he your son?" or "What lovely flowers. Are they from your family?" "I read about that book in the paper. Is it good?"

6. If a client is in pain or is otherwise experiencing discomfort, the nurse should attend to the client's physiological needs first.

Medical/Nursing Vocabulary

abdominal incision: a surgical cut of body tissue in the abdomen

adhere: to stick to or follow

admitting nurse: nurse who admits clients into a hospital

allergic (to): affected by sensitivity to certain substances, which causes an exaggerated or pathological reaction

appendectomy: surgical removal of the appendix (appendix: small tube attached to the beginning of the large intestine, which serves no function but can become infected, causing appendicitis)

assist of 1: with the assistance or help of one person

attending physician: doctor who is in charge of patient care and supervises resident physicians

bathroom privileges: client is allowed to use the bathroom

blood glucose: amount of glucose (sugar) in the blood

clinician: person qualified in the clinical practice of medicine, such as a physician or nurse practitioner

contact precautions: precautions taken to prevent the spread of infection by direct/indirect contact with the client or the client's environment, such as wearing personal protective equipment (PPE), including gown and gloves

diabetes mellitus type 2: a type of diabetes that develops especially in adults and most often in obese individuals, characterized by too much glucose in the blood because of impaired glucose utilization along with impaired insulin production

diagnosis: identifying a disease from its signs and symptoms

fluid balance: the relation between the intake of a particular liquid and its excretion

focused respiratory assessment: an assessment of the respiratory system, including normal and abnormal findings

Full Code: everything is done in the hospital to prolong life (e.g., resuscitation and intubation)

hydration: condition of having adequate fluid in the body tissues

hypertension: abnormally high arterial blood pressure

infection: entry of microbes into the body, which then multiply in the body

insulin: a hormone produced in the pancreas that controls how the body converts sugar into energy and regulates the level of sugar in the blood and that when produced in insufficient quantities results in diabetes mellitus

insulin protocol: standardized plan for administering insulin

Mantoux: intradermal test for tuberculosis that indicates past or present infection

medical/surgical: unit in the hospital for clients requiring treatment for general medical conditions or general surgical procedures

monitor(ed): to check or examine a client's progress

normal saline: a salt solution, made of distilled water and approximately 0.9% solution of sodium chloride, which is introduced into the body intravenously though a drip

positive: shows the presence of something

purulent exudate: yellow liquid composed of blood serum, pieces of dead tissue, white blood cells, and the remains of bacteria, formed by the body in reaction to infection; also called pus

regulate: to fix or adjust the time, amount, degree, or rate of something so that it works in a regular way

site: place where something happened or is located, or where an incision is to be made in an operation

stabilize: to make a condition stable or not changing

stable: not changing or fluctuating

sulfa: synthetic antibiotic derived from the chemical compound sulfanilamide

ulcer: open sore in the skin or mucous membrane, which is inflamed and difficult to heal

vital signs: signs of life, specifically the pulse rate, respiration rate, body temperature, blood pressure, and oxygen saturation of a person

wound consult: consultation with a health care provider who is certified in wound care

▶ Activity 1.3: Dose of Medication

1. ___mg___ milligram
2. ___mL___ milliliter
3. ___mEq___ milliequivalent
4. ___D_5W___ 5% dextrose in water
5. ___g___ gram
6. ___mcg___ microgram
7. ___gtt___ drop

▶ Activity 1.4: Identifying Medication Orders, Labs, Tests, and Nursing Actions in Scenario #1

Medications

Normal saline (NS): Maintains hydration and fluid balance; 0.9% (NS) IV running at 125 mL/hr (0.9% means 9 g of sodium chloride for every 100 L of water)

Enalapril: Stabilizes high blood pressure; 5 mg PO BID

Extra Strength Tylenol: Relieves pain; 500 mg PO PRN q4–6h

Multivitamin tablet: Supplements vitamin and mineral intake; 1 (tablet) PO daily

NPH insulin: Regulates blood sugar; subcut per insulin protocol

Cefazolin: Fights infection; 2 g in D_5W 50 mL IVPB q8h

The additional information that is provided (with the exception of NPH insulin) is as follows: amount of medication, route of medication, and frequency of administration, in that order.

Labs/Tests

chest x-ray

CBC lab

blood glucose capillary sample

Nursing Actions*

Maintain client on diabetic diet

Take vital signs q4h

Take daily weight

Assess incision site

Assess toe ulcer

Assess pain

Perform focused respiratory assessment

Take contact precautions

*Note that consults are not included here as they are not performed by a nurse or nursing assistive personnel (NAP).

▶ Activity 1.5: Plan of Care: Planning for Client's Care

1. Infection secondary to appendectomy
2. Hypertension, diabetes mellitus type 2, right toe ulcer
3. Twice daily: 8:00 a.m. and 8:00 p.m. 12 hours apart. One dose is given during the day shift and one dose during the evening shift.
4. NS (normal saline) and cefazolin
5. VS q4h, daily weight, abdominal incision site, toe ulcer, pain, focused respiratory

Nursing Diagnosis: Thinking Holistically about Mrs. Jackson

The intervention "Nurse will offer client a back rub and teach client relaxation techniques by end of shift" reflects care of Mrs. Jackson's psychosocial need to reduce her anxiety.

▶ Activity 1.6: Nursing Diagnosis: Nursing Interventions and Desired Outcomes

Nursing Intervention	Desired Outcome
1. ____c____ Nurse will offer client a back rub and teach client relaxation techniques by the end of shift.	a. Client will report decreased pain level of 2 (scale 0–10) in abdomen within 1 hour of analgesic administration.
2. ____d____ Nurse will teach client splinting techniques by the end of shift.	b. Client will report decreased pain level of 2 (scale 0–10) in toe ulcer within 1 hour of analgesic administration. .
3. ____a____ Nurse will administer pain medication and a cool pack to relieve abdominal pain during shift.	c. Client will report less anxiety by the end of shift.
4. ____b____ Nurse will clean toe ulcer, apply dressing, and elevate the foot during shift.	d. Client will demonstrate how to splint the abdominal wound by the end of shift.

▶ Activity 1.7: Subjective vs. Objective Data

1. **OBJ** Mr. F has not had a bowel movement in 3 days.
2. **SUBJ** Mr. F complains of being constipated.
3. **SUBJ** Ms. G says she has a pain that comes and goes in her left eye.
4. **OBJ** Both eyelids appear swollen.
5. **OBJ** The wrist looks red.
6. **SUBJ** Mr. K says that the wrist does not hurt when he moves it.
7. **SUBJ** "I forget to take my pills."
8. **SUBJ** "I can't live without sugar in my food."
9. **OBJ** Weight 98 kg (215 lbs); gain of 4.5 kg (10 lbs).
10. **OBJ** Blood pressure 190/100 mm Hg.

▶ Activity 1.8: Identifying Subjective and Objective Data

Subjective Data

Pt stated upon admission, "I feel weak in my knees and this toe ulcer is driving me crazy. I can barely feel my foot now and sometimes the pain is unbearable!"

5 pt rated pain at incision site at 5 and toe pain at 10 on 0–10 scale.

Objective Data

Area around incision is warm to touch and slightly red.

Right toe is swollen and contains purulent exudate.

▶ Activity 1.9: Understanding Telephone Order Report

1. Cefazolin
2. Vancomycin and ibuprofen
3. Mrs. Jackson is given both vancomycin and ibuprofen immediately.
4. Mrs. Jackson's vitals are taken every 30 minutes now. In Scenario #1, they were taken every 4 hours. Because of the dehiscence at the abdominal incision site and the risk of a worsening infection, the nurse needs to check Mrs. Jackson's vitals more often until the client is stable again—that is, until the client's vital signs are normal and there is no bleeding.
5. Mrs. Jackson is given 400 mg of ibuprofen now. In Scenario #1, she was given 500 mg of Extra Strength Tylenol, as needed. Because of the increase in pain and likely inflammation that Mrs. Jackson is experiencing from the dehiscence at the abdominal incision site, she is given 1 dose of ibuprofen, as it has anti-inflammatory properties. After that, the nurse will continue with the order for Tylenol, as needed.
6. Mrs. Jackson is put on bed rest to decrease abdominal pressure in order to prevent reoccurrence of the dehiscence and thereby promote healing of the incision site. In addition, limiting the client's movements may help alleviate the pain that she is experiencing and prevent more pain from occurring.

▶ Activity 1.10: Providing Holistic Care

The client's anxiety secondary to the dehiscence of her abdominal wound is identified as one of the problems in the progress note. In addition, a reduction in the client's anxiety is listed as one of the desired outcomes in the care of the client. Specific ways to address the client's anxiety in the plan of care include teaching the client about wound care and splinting techniques, as well as about relaxation techniques, and providing a quiet, healing environment for the client. The client is also encouraged to inform the nurse about any concerns she has regarding her health and care. In addition, the client's health status and progress continue to be monitored and medications administered per MAR, the client is maintained on bed rest, the client is turned every couple of hours, and the client is encouraged to drink fluids. In sum, the client's anxiety is addressed at both the psychosocial and physiological levels. In addition, the attending physician has updated the client's husband about her progress, the husband is included in a discussion about the client's plan of care, and the client is provided with opportunities to spend time with her children, all reflecting a holistic perspective of the client as a member of a family system.

▶ Activity 1.11: Understanding the 24-Hour Clock

12-Hour Clock	24-Hour Clock
1. 4:40 a.m.	1. 0440
2. 4:40 p.m.	2. 1640
3. 10:10 a.m.	3. 1010
4. 10:10 p.m.	4. 2210
5. 12:30 a.m.	5. 0030
6. 12:30 p.m.	6. 1230

▶ Activity 1.12: Understanding the Metric System

Household Measurement		Metric Measurement
1.	c half a cup	a. 5.0 cm in diameter
2.	a 2 inches in diameter	b. 90 g
3.	g 4 inches	c. 125 mL
4.	h 11 pounds	d. 1500 mL
5.	f 2 fluid ounces	e. 30 mL
6.	e 2 tablespoons	f. 60 mL
7.	b 3 ounces	g. 10 cm in diameter
8.	d 3 pints	h. 5 kg

▶ Activity 1.13: Analyzing Effectiveness of Communication

Note: Answers will vary and will not yet reflect an understanding of therapeutic communication skills.

1. Mrs. Jackson is most concerned that she is not getting any better. Indeed, her medical issues seem to be increasing, and in the process she has become tired and discouraged.

2. The nurse asks Mrs. Jackson questions and shows that she is interested in her.

3. Yes, the nurse gives Mrs. Jackson information that should be reassuring. She also shows that she cares and gives Mrs. Jackson a chance to talk about what is on her mind.

4. At the end of the interview, the nurse could have asked about Mrs. Jackson's family. Mrs. Jackson might have appreciated her expression of interest and the opportunity to talk about her family, especially her children.

▶ Activity 1.14: Analyzing Dialog for Empathy and Attending Behaviors

1. The nurse notices that Mrs. Jackson seems upset and asks her what is going on. She listens to what Mrs. Jackson tells her and asks follow-up questions. The nurse also speaks openly about feelings. She says to Mrs. Jackson that Mrs. Jackson seems upset and later in the dialog, the nurse acknowledges how challenging the situation has been for Mrs. Jackson. The nurse also invites Mrs. Jackson to ask any other questions or bring up any concerns she has.

2. By recognizing and acknowledging Mrs. Jackson's feelings, the nurse validates those feelings, thereby demonstrating empathy toward Mrs. Jackson. By encouraging Mrs. Jackson to talk about her feelings and concerns, the nurse demonstrates openness toward the client and fosters trust in their relationship.

3. By asking several questions about the toe ulcer, providing information about the dehiscence, and acknowledging the client's feelings, the nurse addresses both the client's physiological and psychosocial needs.

4. The nurse has created trust between herself and Mrs. Jackson, as Mrs. Jackson opens up about her deepest concern: that she is not getting any better and in the process has become tired and discouraged.

5. As soon as she realizes that Mrs. Jackson is upset about something, the nurse sits down to be at the same eye level as Mrs. Jackson. She moves her chair close to Mrs. Jackson and leans in so she can easily hear what Mrs. Jackson says in response to her question about what is going on. She asks follow-up questions that show she has been listening to Mrs. Jackson and squats to visually inspect the toe that has been bothering Mrs. Jackson.

▶ Activity 1.15: Analyzing "I" Statements

"You" statements by the nurse could be interpreted by the client as judgmental and provoke a defensive or evasive response by the client. A more effective way of finding out why the client did not eat anything is for the nurse to use an "I" statement. With an "I" statement, the nurse simply states an observation in a neutral way, without judging the client. In response, the client is more likely to tell the nurse what is bothering him or her. "I" statements encourage a more open, thus more accurate, exchange of information between the nurse and client.

In the dialog, the nurse states, "I see that you seem upset" when the nurse enters the room and notices that Mrs. Jackson seems upset. Rather than state, "You seem upset," which could provoke a defensive reaction by the client, the nurse simply states what she observes and also uses the verb "seem," which indicates possibility, not certainty.

Later the nurse states, "I will take a closer look [at the toe] shortly." Toward the end of the interaction, the nurse says, "I understand that it has been quite challenging for you…" and "I just want to let you know that… my team and I will do our very best to care for you." The latter examples reflect other uses of "I" statements–that is, to provide verbal reassurance to the client and to explain to the client a procedure that the nurse is preparing to do.

▶ Activity 1.16: Using "I" Statements

Ineffective Statement	Effective "I" Statement
1. "Mr. Nguyen, you should get ready for your bath now."	1. "Mr. Nguyen, I'd like you to get ready for your bath now."
2. "You frequently miss your appointments."	2. "I notice that you have missed several appointments. Is something the matter?"
3. "You haven't eaten anything on your plate."	3. "I see that you did not eat anything. How are you feeling?"
4. "You are not very clear."	4. "I did not understand you. Can you say it again?"
5. "Don't we look nice today."	5. "I think you look nice today."
6. "It's time for us to get ready for your family's visit."	6. "It's time for you to get ready for your family's visit. They'll be here soon."

▶ Activity 1.17: Analyzing Dialog for Reflection

After Mrs. Jackson states, "Well, my problems are getting to be too much," the nurse reflects by saying, "You're concerned about your health," thereby encouraging Mrs. Jackson to continue talking about her concerns and to explore her feelings more deeply. Also, at the end of her description of what she did to make her toe feel better, Mrs. Jackson states, "It's gotten worse." In response, the nurse reflects, by asking, "Your toe is still in pain?" The use of reflection here verbalizes what Mrs. Jackson has implied about her pain, thus acknowledging and validating what the client is experiencing.

▶ Activity 1.18: Using Reflection

Client's Statement	Nurse's Reflection
1. "I don't want to talk about anything. Just go away."	1. "You don't want to talk?" (*with rising intonation*)
2. "I'm so angry with myself."	2. "You're angry?" *(with rising intonation)*
3. "Why do you care? I'm just going to die."	3. "You feel you're going to die?" *(with rising intonation)*
4. (*crying*) "I'll never get better."	4. "You feel you'll never get better?" *(with rising intonation)*
5. (*sadly*) "Nobody cares about me. No one visits me here."	5. "You seem sad."
6. "Nurse, what time is it? The doctor was supposed to be here this morning."	6. "You seem anxious."

▶ Activity 1.19: Considering Use of Reflection

1. Answers will vary, but some students may have difficulty using reflection. They may complain that it sounds unnatural, and they may worry how they can be genuine with a client when they feel unnatural.
2. Answers will vary, but some students may find it difficult to reflect feelings of an intense personal nature, especially related to death and dying.
3. Answers will vary, but some students may find it difficult to use reflection when the client is clearly very upset.
4. Answers will vary, but some nurses and clients may have difficulty talking about feelings if, in their cultures, it is uncommon to do so, especially feelings that are intensely personal, particularly with strangers. There may be other cultural barriers related to age, gender, or ethnicity.

▶ Activity 1.20: Analyzing Dialog for Verbal Reassurance

The nurse reassures Mrs. Jackson that the nurse is listening, that the client's concerns are real and important, and that the nurse understands the client's concerns: "I understand that it has been quite challenging for you with all that you have been going through, and indeed health concerns can be very draining." The nurse also reassures Mrs. Jackson that good care is being given: "I just want to let you know that you are in the right place because my team and I will do our very best to care for you."

Mrs. Jackson seems to relax a bit after the nurse verbally reassures her. She responds with, "I appreciate it." She also goes on to ask the nurse to take it easy with her, revealing some vulnerability on her part. Her willingness to reveal that vulnerability reflects the trust that has been established between the client and nurse.

▶ Activity 1.21: Using Verbal Reassurance

Client's Statement	Nurse's Response
1. "My stroke was weeks ago, and I still haven't recovered. I don't think I'll ever get better."	1. "I know you are concerned, but it can take many months to recover from a stroke. You are making steady progress."
2. "Nobody here cares what happens to me."	2. "I care what happens to you."
3. "I heard on the radio that there is a shortage of nurses at this hospital. What kind of care will I get here after surgery?"	3. "There is a shortage of nurses in many hospitals, so it can take longer to be scheduled for surgery. But once you have surgery, the nurse/client ratio at this hospital meets strict guidelines that are required by the state."
4. "What difference does it make? I'm just a number here anyway."	4. "This is a large hospital, but within each unit, we know our clients by name and care what happens to them."
5. "My foot is in a lot of pain; I can hardly walk. I'm worried that it will never get better."	5. "There has been some trauma to your foot, but ice can be applied to reduce the swelling and that should reduce the pain."
6. "My doctor gave me a prescription for pain medication, but I haven't taken any. I'm concerned I might get addicted."	6. "If you take more medication than you are supposed to, it is possible to become addicted. But it is also important to relieve your body of the pain, so it can focus on healing itself."

▶ Activity 1.22: Analyzing Dialog for Nonverbal Reassurance

The nurse uses a quiet tone of voice when she provides verbal reassurance about the quality of care, and she also places her hand on Mrs. Jackson's shoulder. In this way, she provides nonverbal reassurance that is consistent in message with the verbal reassurance, thereby reinforcing the verbal reassurance and enhancing the nurse/client relationship. Other examples of nonverbal reassurance are listed: the nurse smiles when she enters the room, she leans forward when she first sits down, and she establishes and maintains eye contact when Mrs. Jackson describes her concerns about her toe and abdominal incision.

Through visual, auditory, and kinesthetic means, the nurse provides nonverbal reassurance to Mrs. Jackson that the nurse is listening, the client's concerns are real and important, and the client is being treated like a person. Because the nonverbal reassurance is consistent with the verbal reassurance, the effect is to further relax the client and to strengthen the trust between the client and nurse.

▶ Activity 1.23: Using Nonverbal Reassurance

Client's Statement	Nurse's Response
1. "My stroke was weeks ago, and I still haven't recovered. I don't think I'll ever get better."	1. (*leaning forward; maintaining eye contact*) "I know you are concerned, but it can take many months to recover from a stroke. You are making steady progress."
2. "Nobody here cares what happens to me."	2. (*if standing, putting a hand on the client's shoulder; using a quiet tone of voice*) "I care what happens to you."
3. "I heard on the radio that there is a shortage of nurses at this hospital. What kind of care will I get here after surgery?"	3. (*vocalizing "um-hmm" while listening to the client; using relaxed rate of speech*) "There is a shortage of nurses in many hospitals, so it can take longer to be scheduled for surgery. But once you have surgery, the nurse/client ratio at this hospital meets strict guidelines that are required by the state."
4. "What difference does it make? I'm just a number here anyway."	4. (*if seated, putting a hand on the client's lower arm; maintaining eye contact*) "This is a large hospital, but within each unit, we know our clients by name and care what happens to them."
5. "My foot is in a lot of pain; I can hardly walk. I'm worried that it will never get better."	5. (*nodding head as client talks; looking concerned*) "There has been some damage to your foot, but ice can be applied to reduce the swelling and that should reduce the pain."
6. "My doctor gave me a prescription for pain medication, but I haven't taken any. I'm concerned I might get addicted."	6. (*vocalizing "um-hmm" while listening to the client; maintaining eye contact*) "If you take more medication than you are supposed to, it is possible to become addicted. But it is also important to relieve your body of the pain, so it can focus on healing itself."

Activity 1.24: Analyzing Dialog for Caring Touch

The nurse places her hand on Mrs. Jackson's shoulder while telling Mrs. Jackson that she understands how challenging it has been for her. This example of caring touch provides nonverbal reassurance to the client that the nurse is listening, that the client's concerns are real and important, and, more broadly, that the nurse cares. Nonverbal reassurance reinforces verbal reassurance and enhances the client's trust in the nurse. The nurse uses touch at the end of the interview, rather than at the beginning. Some clients may not wish to be touched, so the nurse waits until trust has been established before she uses touch.

Activity 1.25: Analyzing Dialog for Silence

A moment of silence occurs after the nurse provides Mrs. Jackson with verbal and nonverbal reassurance that the nurse is listening, the client's concerns are real and important, the nurse understands the client's concerns, and good care is being given. It is an emotional moment, as the client has become teary-eyed and revealed her vulnerability. The silence allows the client time to process what the nurse has said and to gather her thoughts. She responds by expressing appreciation to the nurse. The nurse uses silence at the end of the interview, rather than at the beginning. During the portion of the interaction when the nurse is gathering information about the client's concerns, silence might have been misunderstood by the client as the nurse not listening.

Activity 1.26: Considering Cultural Differences in Nonverbal Communication

1–4: Answers will vary.

Activity 1.27: Considering Cultural Differences in the Use of Touch

1–3: Answers will vary.

4. For procedural touch, the nurse should ask the client for permission to touch him and her, and then explain how the procedure will be done and why the procedure is important. For caring touch, permission is generally not asked, as it is something more spontaneous. A nurse should get a sense for a client's degree of comfort with caring touch early in the process of caring for the client and then use caring touch selectively and appropriately with the client, given the client's age, gender, and cultural background, as well as any religious restrictions and the client's medical condition. Nurses should be especially aware of these differences with culturally diverse clients, as they may be more or less comfortable with caring touch.

5. Practicing the use of touch, in particular caring touch, in role plays is one way for nursing students to become comfortable with touch. Videos regarding nurse/client interaction can also show students who are reluctant to use caring touch both how caring touch can be beneficial to clients, as well as how it can be used in certain situations. Eventually, with enough practice, the use of caring touch will become more or less automatic. Procedural touch can be practiced during labs, increasingly with the use of manikins.

Activity 1.28: Considering Cultural Differences in the Use of Silence

1–4: Answers will vary.

Considering Complementary and Alternative Medicine

2

Learning Objectives

- Considering complementary and alternative medicine
- Understanding language clients use to describe symptoms and feelings
- Learning medical/nursing abbreviations related to medication orders: Route of administration
- Identifying medication orders, labs, tests, and nursing actions
- Understanding the language of nursing diagnoses: Statement of problem
- Documenting client care: Using medical/nursing terminology and precise wording
- Avoiding blocks to therapeutic communication: Giving advice, expressing disapproval, judging the client, and false reassurance
- Recognizing cultural differences in blocks to therapeutic communication

Scenario #2

Client: African female, 47 yo

Diagnosis: Exacerbation of COPD (chronic obstructive pulmonary disease) and urinary tract infection

History: Degenerative joint disease, hypertension, COPD

Ms. Yemi Achu is a 47-year-old Ghanaian woman who was admitted to med/surg **diagnosed** with **exacerbation** of COPD (**chronic obstructive pulmonary disease**) and a UTI (**urinary tract infection**). She has a history of DJD (**degenerative joint disease**), HTN (hypertension), and COPD. Upon admission, her RR was 12/min and O_2 sats were 88%, and she reported an increase in coughing and **sputum** production and tightness in the chest. She is anxious about her condition. Ms. Achu has smoked for 25 years. She has tried to quit several times, using a **nicotine patch** and **nicotine gum**, but was not successful. She is Full Code. She is allergic to codeine. The attending physician ordered O_2 at 2 L via NC (**nasal cannula**) to increase oxygen blood level because her O_2 sats fell below 90%. She is on continuous O_2 monitoring with a **pulse oximeter**. Other medications ordered are albuterol 2 puffs BID to **dilate** the **bronchi**, 0.9% NS IV running at 75 mL/hr to maintain hydration and fluid balance, acetaminophen 325–650 mg PO PRN to relieve pain, lisinopril 20 mg PO daily to stabilize high blood pressure, prednisone 10 mg PO BID to reduce the **inflammation**, and gentamicin 70 mg IVPB q8h to fight the infection. Her HOB (head of bed) needs to be raised at least 30° in a **semi-Fowler's position. Vitals** should be assessed q8h. **Passive range of motion** (ROM) should be performed. She is on a low **sodium** (Na^+) diet. A CBC lab has been ordered as well as a **urine culture and sensitivity.** Pt also needs focused respiratory and musculoskeletal assessments. **Pulmonary** and **orthopedic consults** have been ordered. Pt came in with **herbal supplements** that she takes for "energy" at home, but they are not being given to her in the hospital. She is a tailor and is well established in her business. Her niece, nephew, and aunt brought her to the emergency room. Her **primary nurse practitioner** also called to get an update on her progress.

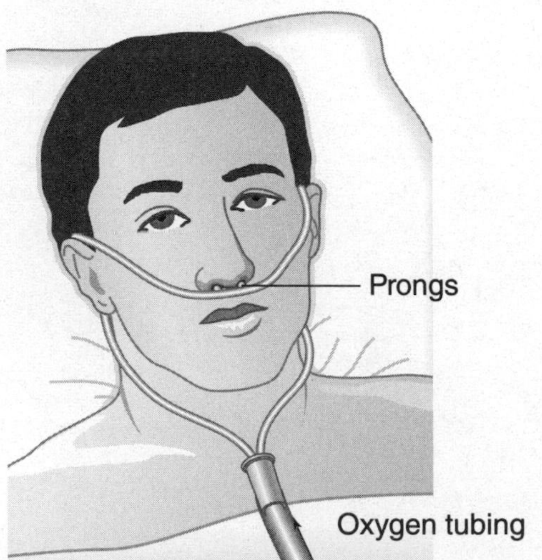

Figure 2-1: Nasal Cannula

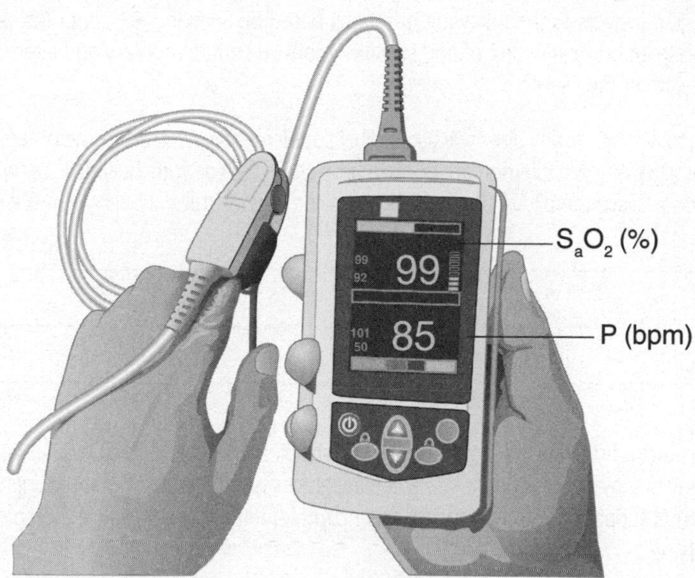

Figure 2-2: Pulse Oximeter

Critical Thinking Skills: Complementary and Alternative Medicine

According to the National Center for Complementary and Alternative Medicine (NCCAM), complementary and alternative medicine (CAM) refers to a wide range of therapies, products, and practices that are used in response to illness but that are not generally considered part of conventional or biomedical medicine. (Source: "Complementary, Alternative, or Integrative Health: What's In a Name?" National Center for Complementary and Alternative Medicine. Available online. URL: http://nccam.nih.gov/whatiscam. Posted on May 13, 2013.) Examples include acupuncture, yoga, meditation, massage, biofeedback, aromatherapy, and the use of supplements. **Alternative medicine** refers to the use of such treatments instead of conventional medicine. **Complementary medicine** refers to their use in addition to conventional medicine. Some treatments have been more rigorously tested than others to determine their efficacy; some are now offered in hospitals and a few are even covered by insurance plans.

Traditional medicine, sometimes referred to as *folk medicine*, is a type of alternative therapy based on the beliefs and practices of a particular cultural group to prevent and treat illness. These practices are generally passed down from one generation to another and are often associated with religious beliefs and rituals, particularly around birth and death. In some cultures traditional medicine involves herbs, plants, minerals, and animal substances. In other cultures, it involves the use of charms, holy words, and rituals. Some people first try traditional medicine before they seek professional health care, especially if there is a language barrier or the perception that the "Western" or biomedical health care system does not meet their needs. Traditional healers not only speak the same language, but they also share the same values and beliefs about health and illness as the client, charge less money, and are more easily accessible than professional health care providers.

As discussed in Chapter One, holistic nursing provides care for all dimensions of the individual, including the physiological, psychosocial, and spiritual. In addition, some hospitals offer complementary and alternative therapies. It is important for nurses to discuss with clients their use of complementary and alternative medicine, as well as their use of traditional medicine.

▶ Activity 2.1: Considering Complementary and Alternative Medicine

Determine your answers to the following questions based on Scenario #2 about Ms. Achu. How would you incorporate an understanding of and sensitivity toward complementary and alternative therapies in your holistic care of the client?

1. According to Ms. Achu, why does she take herbal supplements? What are some other possible reasons? Do you practice any complementary or alternative therapies for your health? If so, what are they, and why do you practice them? Are these practices related to your cultural background? If so, in what ways?

___

___

___

2. Why is Ms. Achu not allowed to take her herbal supplements in the hospital? Do you agree with this policy? Why or why not? Are there some circumstances when it would be appropriate to allow a client to take herbal supplements or to practice other complementary or alternative therapies in the hospital? If so, explain.

___

___

___

3. How is smoking viewed in your culture, particularly for women? How should the nurse approach the issue of smoking with Ms. Achu? How would a nurse in your culture respond to a client who smokes? (For discussion of personal health-related issues, see section on giving advice later in this chapter.)

___

___

___

Understanding and Using Language Effectively in Health Care Settings

The language used in health care settings is different from general, conversational English. Nurses must use medical/nursing terminology as well as specialized ways of communicating with clients. In addition, nurses must understand the language that clients use in the health care setting.

Client Talk: Describing Symptoms and Feelings

Clients use a variety of words and expressions to describe how they are feeling. Many of these words and expressions are colloquial and idiomatic. You may not find them in a standard English dictionary and they cannot be understood word for word. If English is your second language, keep a list of expressions you hear that you do not understand and ask a friend or colleague who is a native speaker of English or an experienced nurse what they mean. To communicate effectively with clients and colleagues, you need to understand spoken, idiomatic English. With time, you may even start to use the same words and expressions.

▶ Activity 2.2: Understanding Client Talk—Describing Symptoms and Feelings

What do the following expressions spoken by Ms. Achu in the Dialog between Nurse and Ms. Achu mean? Write down your understanding of each expression.

1. "I can't seem to catch my breath." ______________________
2. "I wish I had kicked the habit." ______________________
3. "On top of it all…" ______________________
4. "I just don't think I can cope anymore." ______________________

What do the following additional expressions mean? Write down your understanding of each expression.

5. "Sometimes I have dizzy spells." ______________________
6. "I have a splitting headache." ______________________
7. "I took a turn for the worse." ______________________
8. "I was out cold." ______________________

Match the definition with each expression or idiom about how the client is feeling. Write the letter of the definition in the correct blank.

Idiom	Definition
I feel:	
9. ________ down in the dumps	a. not well
10. ________ on top of the world	b. disconnected, disoriented
11. ________ run down	c. better, improving, healing
12. ________ under the weather	d. terrible
13. ________ on the mend	e. nauseous
14. ________ out of it	f. sad
15. ________ blue	g. very good
16. ________ sick to my stomach	h. tired, without energy
17. ________ like shit	i. depressed

Medical/Nursing Vocabulary

How many of the bolded medical/nursing words used in Scenario #2 about Ms. Achu do you already know? For those words you do not know, look them up in a nursing textbook, an English-language medical dictionary, or online resources. Refer to the definitions in the Answer Key for Chapter Two, as needed.

Medical/Nursing Abbreviations

Identify as many of the abbreviations from Scenario #2 about Ms. Achu as you can. Refer, as needed, to the list of Medical/Nursing Abbreviations in the Appendix.

Expansion of Medical/Nursing Abbreviations: Medication Orders (Route of Administration)

The medications that Ms. Achu is currently taking are included in Scenario #2. Abbreviations and acronyms are commonly used in medication orders.

Medication Orders

There are 7 parts to a medication order. (See the Medication Orders section in Chapter One to review the 7 parts.) In Chapter One, you were introduced to dose, the fourth part. Route of administration is the fifth part.

▶ Activity 2.3: Route of Administration

Write the correct abbreviation for each word or phrase used in medication orders in the blank provided. The first one has been done for you.

ID gtt IM PO R subcut IV MDI

1. ___PO___ by mouth
2. __________ subcutaneous
3. __________ intradermal
4. __________ intramuscular
5. __________ intravenous
6. __________ drop
7. __________ metered dose inhaler

8 __________ rectally

Expansion of Scenario #2: Understanding Medication Orders, Labs, Tests, and Nursing Actions

When Ms. Achu is admitted to the hospital, she is assessed by the attending physician, who orders medications, labs (laboratory tests), and other tests for her. In addition, both the physician and the nurse who is assigned to care for Ms. Achu on the medical-surgical unit determine appropriate nursing actions. Some of these nursing care actions are carried out by the nurse; some are carried out by the licensed practical or vocational nurse (LPN/LVN) or nursing assistive personnel (NAP); and some are carried out by other health care professionals.

▶ Activity 2.4: Identifying Medication Orders, Labs, Tests, and Nursing Actions in Scenario #2

Write down the medications that are ordered for Ms. Achu. Why is each medication ordered? What information is provided for each medication, and in what order? For each medication, write the information that is provided.

Medications

Write down the labs and other tests that have been ordered and the nursing actions that have been planned for Ms. Achu.

Labs/Tests

Nursing Actions

Expansion of Scenario #2: Plan of Care

When nursing students prepare for clinical, they often use forms like the Plan of Care (Figure 2-1) to record essential information about the client from the client's record and to plan for the client's care. Note that the route of medication is not always specified on the Plan of Care, as nurses would refer to the MAR (Medical Administration Record) before administering medications. This Plan of Care reflects care for Ms. Achu during the day shift on her first day in the hospital. The vital signs recorded were taken at the beginning of the shift.

Figure 2-3: Plan of Care
Scenario #2

ROOM	**DIET**	**OTHER**	**T**	**P**	**RR**	**BP**
2394	Low Na^+ diet	Full Code HOB in semi-Fowler's position Acetaminophen 325–650 mg PO PRN	98.4	87	18	140/94
INITIALS YA	**ACTIVITY** Passive ROM		**O_2 sats** 92% RA*			
Dx Exacerbation of COPD UTI	**IVs** 0.9% NS at 75 mL/hr Gentamicin 70 mg PB q8h		**NOTES**			
MHx DJD HTN COPD	**LABS/TESTS/APPTS** CBC Urine culture and sensitivity Pulmonary consult Orthopedic consult	**ASSESSMENTS** VS q8h Continuous O_2 sat monitoring Focused respiratory Focused musculoskeletal				
MDs Dr. Mahmood						
TREATMENTS O_2 at 2L via NC if O_2 sats fall below 90%						
ALLERGY Codeine	**PAIN**		**OUTPUTS** N/A			

0700/1900	**0800/2000**	**0900/2100**	**1000/2200**	**1100/1300**	**1200/2400**
Lisinopril 20 mg	Albuterol 2 puffs Prednisone 10 mg				
1300/0100	**1400/0200**	**1500/0300**	**1600/0400**	**1700/0500**	**1800/0600**

*RA (room air) = that is, regular conditions of breathing, without any added oxygen

▶ Activity 2.5: Plan of Care: Planning for Client's Care

Answer the following questions with information that is provided in the Plan of Care regarding Ms. Achu.

1. What is Ms. Achu's diagnosis?

____

____

2. What is Ms. Achu's medical history?

____

____

3. How often and when is Ms. Achu given 2 puffs albuterol?

____

____

4. What medications does Ms. Achu receive intravenously?

____

____

5. What assessments are planned for Ms. Achu?

____

____

Nursing Diagnosis: Planning Holistic Care for Ms. Achu

Based on the information provided in the client's record and the nurse's assessment* of the client, the nurse writes a nursing diagnosis and a goal for treating the client. The nurse also identifies nursing interventions and desired outcomes to accomplish that goal. In planning holistic care for Ms. Achu, the nurse identifies interventions that address Ms. Achu's psychosocial and spiritual needs, as well as her physiologic needs. Review the interventions in Activity 2.6. Which nursing intervention reflects care of Ms. Achu's psychosocial needs?

Nursing Diagnosis: Impaired spontaneous ventilation related to fluid overload and respiratory muscle fatigue as manifested by 88% O_2 sats, increase in cough and sputum production, and chest tightness.

Goal: Client will have adequate energy level and muscle function to maintain spontaneous breathing.

*A physical assessment is usually conducted when a client is first admitted to the hospital, either a head-to-toe assessment or a focused assessment on a specific problem area, followed by a head-to-toe assessment, as needed. Information from this assessment is included in the client's record and is reviewed by the nurse caring for Ms. Achu.

▶ Activity 2.6: Nursing Diagnosis: Nursing Interventions and Desired Outcomes

Match each Desired Outcome for Ms. Achu with the corresponding Nursing Intervention. Write the letter of the Desired Outcome in the correct blank.

Nursing Intervention	Desired Outcome
1. __________ Nurse will teach client huff coughing* technique by the end of shift.	a. Client will report less fatigue from breathing by the end of shift.
2. __________ Nurse will keep head of bed elevated above 30 degrees, encourage use of incentive spirometer,† and assess client's breathing and oxygen saturation throughout shift.	b. O_2 saturation will improve to 90% by the end of shift.
3. __________ Nurse will administer inhaler medications as ordered and provide mouth care after inhalers during shift.	c. Client will report less anxiety by the end of shift.
4. __________ Nurse will offer hand massage to enhance relaxation and decrease anxiety‡ by the end of shift.	d. Client will have decreased crackles heard over lung fields within an hour of treatment.

*In huff coughing, the client opens the glottis and says the word "huff" during exhalation.

†Incentive spirometer is a device that measures the flow of air inhaled through the mouthpiece; clients are encouraged to use it to improve their ventilation.

‡Hand massaging will also have the physiological effects of decreasing oxygen demand and increasing oxygen perfusion.

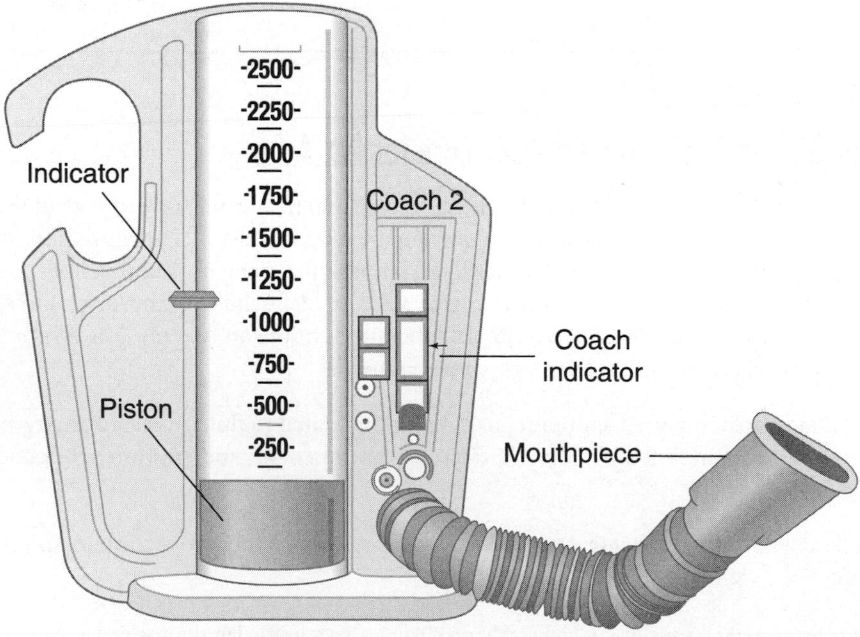

Figure 2-4: Incentive Spirometer

Expansion of Nursing Diagnosis: Understanding the Language of Nursing Diagnoses (Statement of Problem)

Nursing diagnoses are statements about the client's response to illness. They are very different from medical diagnoses, which concern the disease process itself. Clients vary in their responses to illness, whereas disease processes are fairly uniform from one client to another. In addition, nursing diagnoses can change as the client's response to illness changes, but the medical diagnosis remains fairly constant as long as the disease process is present.

Nursing diagnoses also consider the client in a holistic manner, or as a whole person. They address physiological responses to disease, as well as psychological, sociocultural, and spiritual responses. Students are generally expected to identify both physiological and psychosocial nursing diagnoses in their care plan. Actual nursing diagnoses describe the client's response to health conditions or life processes and are based on the nurse's assessment. Risk diagnoses describe the clients responses to health conditions or life processes that may develop. Health promotion diagnoses describe the clients readiness to change behaviors to improve health. For example:

Medical Diagnosis	**Nursing Diagnoses**
Myocardial infarction	Activity intolerance related to decreased cardiac output (physiological response)
	Ineffective coping (psychological response)
	Interrupted family processes (sociocultural response)
	Death anxiety (spiritual response)

Most nursing diagnoses consist of 3 parts:

1. **Problem (P):** Statement of the client's response to the illness or health condition
2. **Etiology (E):** Factors that contribute to or probable causes of the client's response
3. **Signs and symptoms (S):** Defining characteristics or cluster of signs and symptoms of the problem that the client exhibits

Problem (P)

The first part of a diagnosis states the Problem or the client's response to the illness. The Problem is taken from a taxonomy or set of diagnostic labels established by the North American Nursing Diagnosis Association (NANDA). The purpose of this taxonomy is to standardize the language of nursing care. Standardized nursing language provides clear, precise, and consistent terminology that nurses can use to refer to the same clinical problems and treatments.

Examples of problems:	Constipation
	Ineffective breastfeeding

Risk Diagnoses

Some diagnoses are actual or present at the time of the assessment and are referred to as *actual diagnoses.* By contrast, *risk diagnoses* describe the client's response to health conditions or life processes that may develop in the future. Compare the following examples:

Actual diagnosis:	Activity intolerance **Definition:** When the client does not have enough physiological or psychological energy to complete daily activities
Risk diagnosis:	Risk for activity intolerance **Definition:** When the client is at risk for not having enough physiological or psychological energy to complete required daily activities

Health Promotion Diagnoses

Diagnoses that are associated with the quality or state of being healthy, rather than a disease process, are referred to as *health promotion diagnoses.* These diagnoses consist of the NANDA label only. Some *health promotion* diagnoses begin with the words *readiness for enhanced. Enhance* means "to make greater, to increase in quality, to attain a more desired state, or to increase well-being."

Examples of health promotion diagnoses:	Effective breastfeeding Readiness for enhanced parenting

Use of *Specify* in Nursing Diagnoses

Some diagnostic labels are followed by the word *specify* to indicate that additional information is needed. The nurse must specify the kind of knowledge that is deficient or the behavior that is healthy or the diagnosis will be too general, as in the following examples:

Deficient knowledge (specify): __________	Deficient knowledge: cognitive deficits
Health-seeking behaviors (specify): __________	Health-seeking behaviors: low-fat diet

Use of Qualifiers in Nursing Diagnoses

Qualifiers or adjectives are sometimes used in nursing diagnoses. The most common are *impaired* and *ineffective*, as in the following examples:

Examples:	Impaired physical mobility Ineffective breastfeeding

▶ Activity 2.7: Understanding Qualifiers

Match each qualifier with its definition. Write the qualifier in the correct blank.

Qualifiers

compromised	disabled	impaired
decreased	disturbed	ineffective
deficient	dysfunctional	interrupted
delayed	imbalanced	perceived

Definitions

1. ______________________ limited or unable
2. ______________________ not sufficient in degree, amount, or quality
3. ______________________ to break the continuity of a process
4. ______________________ out of balance or proportion
5. ______________________ to become aware of through use of the senses
6. ______________________ made vulnerable to threat of infection or injury
7. ______________________ not producing the desired or intended effect
8. ______________________ slow, late, or postponed
9. ______________________ agitated; interrupted
10. ______________________ functioning that is abnormal
11. ______________________ smaller in degree, size, or amount
12. ______________________ weakened, damaged, reduced

▶ Activity 2.8: Identifying Qualifiers in Diagnostic Statements

Review the Nursing Diagnosis for Ms. Achu. Identify the qualifier that is used and write it in the space provided.

Qualifiers

____

Telephone Report

Nurses sometimes contact the clinician by telephone about a client—for example, when there is a medical emergency or when there is a significant or noteworthy change in the client's condition.

The nurse caring for Ms. Achu contacts the attending physician by telephone about a change in Ms. Achu's condition. Here is what the nurse reports to the physician, referred to as a *telephone report*:

> *Hello, Dr. Mahmood. This is Debra Ventura, the RN caring for Ms. Achu, a 47-year-old woman, in Room 2394. She was admitted for an exacerbation of COPD and has a UTI. She has a history of degenerative joint disease, hypertension, and COPD. She is on 2 liters of oxygen and has a normal saline IV running at 75 milliliters per hour. Her O_2 sats are currently at 84% and RR 12. Her breathing is distressed and she is short of breath. She is using her accessory muscles and is wheezing on inspiration and crackles heard over lung fields during expiration. She took her albuterol puffs 30 minutes ago, but there has not been significant improvement. The respiratory therapist gave her budesonide via a nebulizer* right before the albuterol puffs. Her blood pressure is 150 over 100. She complains of stiffness in her neck and elbow joints. Her output has decreased and her urine is still nebulous. I suspect that she has fluid overload that is causing her decrease in oxygen and consequently shortness of breath. How would you like us to proceed with her care?*

*nebulizer = a device used to administer medication in the form of mist inhaled into the lungs

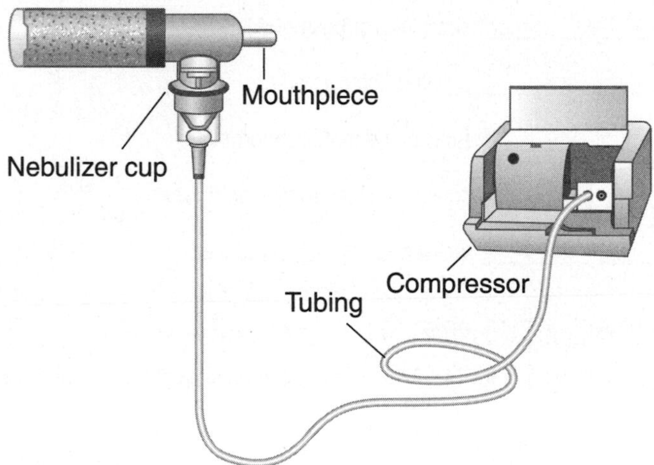

Figure 2-5: Nebulizer

Documentation of Telephone Report

After completing the telephone report, the nurse documents the date, the time, the person called, the person who received the information, what information was given, and what information was received. Figure 2-2 shows the documentation of the telephone report about Ms. Achu.

Figure 2-6: Documentation of Telephone Report

08-17-13 0830 Debra Ventura. Distressed breathing and SOB. O_2 sats 84% and RR 12. Wheezing and crackles heard over lung fields. On O_2 at 2 L. No improvement post albuterol puffs. BP 150/100. Stiffness in neck and elbow joints and decreased urine output. Dr. Mahmood notified via phone.
--D. Ventura, RN

Telephone Order

In response to telephone reports, clinicians usually change medication and other orders for the client. Here is the attending physician's response to the nurse's report about Ms. Achu, referred to as a *telephone order* (T.O.). Note that spoken delivery of medication orders differs in some ways from written orders.

> *Hello, Debra. From your brief summary on Ms. Achu in Room 2394, increase her oxygen to 4 liters. Administer 12 micrograms of formoterol powder using a dry powder inhaler once and 2 puffs of beclomethasone every 6 hours. Elevate head of bed to 45 degrees. Stop the normal saline IV, saline lock the IV, and start her on 20 milligrams of Lasix* IV push once. Strictly monitor her input and output as Lasix will increase her urine output. Monitor her blood pressure every 20 minutes for the next hour and update me. From there, I will be able to better determine if an anti-hypertensive medication should be administered. Also, encourage her to use her incentive spirometer every 2 hours to prevent fluid accumulation in her lungs and possible pneumonia. For the stiffness in her neck and elbows, give her 800 milligrams of metaxalone now and another dose in 6 hours. Assess the stiffness in 2 hours and update me. Continue with the gentamicin 70 milligrams IVPB every 8 hours, as it will help with the UTI. I will see her when I do my evening rounds. Thank you.*

*The generic name for this medication is furosemide, but the brand name Lasix is also used frequently in the clinical setting.

Documentation of Telephone Order

The nurse must document telephone orders from the clinician. Figure 2-3 shows the nurse's documentation of the telephone order about Ms. Achu, referred to as a *telephone order report.*

Figure 2-7: Telephone Order Report

1. Increase O_2 via NC to 4 L
2. Administer formoterol 12 mcg inhaler once
3. Administer beclomethasone 2 puffs q6h
4. Administer metaxalone 800 mg PO stat and in 6h
5. Continue to administer gentamicin 70 mg IVPB q8h
6. D/C NS IV
7. Start Lasix 20 mg IV push once
8. Strictly monitor I&O
9. Elevate HOB to 45°
10. Monitor BP q20 min for 1 hr and update MD
11. Encourage use of incentive spirometer q2h
12. Assess stiffness in neck and elbows in 2h and notify MD

08-17-13 0850

T.O. from Dr. Mahmood/Debra Ventura, RN

▶ Activity 2.9: Understanding Telephone Order Report

Answer the following questions based on the telephone order report about Ms. Achu.

1. Which medication for Ms. Achu is discontinued?

___

___

2. What new medications are ordered for Ms. Achu?

___

___

3. How much and when is Ms. Achu given metaxalone?

___

___

4. Why is Ms. Achu encouraged to use the incentive spirometer?

___

___

5. How high should Ms. Achu's HOB be elevated? How high is the HOB in Scenario #2? Why is there a difference in the height of the HOB, do you think?

___

___

6. How much oxygen does the physician order for Ms. Achu? How much is ordered for her in Scenario #2? Why is there a difference in the amount of oxygen, do you think?

____

____

Documentation of Client Care: Progress Note

At the end of the shift, the nurse documents the care that was given to the client in the form of a progress note. Here is the progress note about the care that was provided to Ms. Achu.

Progress Note

Identify Problem(s)

Respiratory distress, stiffness of neck and elbow joints, fluid overload, elevated blood pressure, cloudy urine, anxiety secondary to SOB

Desired Outcome(s)

Pt will report decreased shortness of breath within 15 minutes of oxygen therapy.

Pt will report increased comfort in the neck and elbow joints within 1 hour of analgesic administration.

Lungs will be clear to auscultation by the end of shift.

Blood pressure will return to preadmission values by the end of shift.

Urine will be less cloudy by the end of antibiotic therapy.

Pt will report less anxiety by the end of shift.

Evaluation

VSS stable except BP 150/100. MD notified of BP, and MD stopped NS IV and started Lasix as initial intervention to decrease BP and fluid overload. Pt c/o stiffness of neck and elbow joints. MD notified, and metaxalone 800 mg ordered. 1st dose administered at 1015; next due 6 hours after 1st dose. Pt on O_2 at 4 L via nasal cannula. Pt on low sodium diet and eats 75% of meals. Passive ROM done 4 times daily. Pt denied nausea and vomiting, and her bowel sounds are active. SOB makes her slightly nervous, but after nebulizer she calms down and reports sleeping well. Urine was still cloudy during last assessment, so pt continues to receive gentamicin IVPB. O_2 sats increased to 92%. Her niece and nephew are supportive, and nurse practitioner updated on progress.

Plan

Continue to monitor client health status and progress. Continue to administer medications per MAR. Continue with passive ROM. RT will continue to administer respiratory meds via nebulizer. Encourage pt to use incentive spirometer q2h and assess progress. Teach pt importance of smoking cessation. Provide quiet, healing environment and music therapy for pt and continue with hand massage to promote well-being. Discuss plan of care with pt and family, as well as nurse practitioner. Encourage pt to inform nurse of any concerns regarding her health and care.

▶ Activity 2.10: Providing Holistic Care

Determine your answers to the following questions based on the care provided to Ms. Achu.

1. How does the plan (of care) in the progress note reflect holistic care of Ms. Achu? How have Ms. Achu's psychosocial and physiological needs been addressed in the plan?

___

___

___

___

___

2. Are any complementary or alternative therapies included in the plan (of care) for Ms. Achu? If so, what are they?

___

___

Expansion of Documentation of Client Care: Characteristics of Effective Documentation

To document accurately and effectively, use medical/nursing terminology and other precise words and expressions.

Medical/Nursing Terminology

Use medical/nursing terminology that exactly and precisely describes medical conditions, not terms used by the general public. For example, rather than *went to the bathroom,* use *voided.*

▶ Activity 2.11: Understanding Medical/Nursing Terminology

Match the medical/nursing terms with the corresponding layperson's terms. Write the letter of the medical/nursing term in the correct blank. The first one has been done for you.

Medical/Nursing Terminology

a. palpitations
b. anorectic
c. radiate
d. intermittent pain
e. serous drainage
f. abduct
g. diaphoretic
h. voided
i. tingling
j. edema
k. sanguineous drainage
l. substernal
m. flex
n. brown fluid
o. copious
p. epistaxis
q. clear fluid
r. dyspneic
s. expels flatus
t. at rest
u. has full ROM
v. marked pallor
w. wet pack
x. emesis

Layperson's Terms

1. ___h___ went to the bathroom
2. __________ move
3. __________ bend
4. __________ under the breast
5. __________ spread out
6. __________ sweating
7. __________ pins and needles
8. __________ abnormally rapid or irregular heart beat
9. __________ no appetite
10. __________ yellowish liquid (from wound)
11. __________ bloody liquid (from wound)
12. __________ pain that comes and goes
13. __________ swelling
14. __________ very pale
15. __________ has difficulty breathing
16. __________ when resting
17. __________ wet towel
18. __________ is able to move wrist
19. __________ bloody nose
20. __________ vomiting
21. __________ passes a lot of gas
22. __________ water-like liquid
23. __________ brownish liquid
24. __________ large amount

Precise Wording

Record factual information that is based on observation and assessment of the client's current health problems and care provided. Be exact or precise in your choice of words and provide specific details. Avoid general words, such as "abnormal" or "large," which can be interpreted in different ways. For example, *abnormal breathing* does not state in what way the breathing is abnormal. *Resp shallow, irregular* is more precise.

General: abnormal breathing

Precise: *resp shallow, irregular*

Use medical/nursing terminology and include all relevant details, such as size and duration, to describe the condition. For example, instead of "nosebleed," use "*epistaxis. 1 min duration. Sm amt sanguineous drainage.*"

General: nosebleed

Precise: *Epistaxis. 1 min duration. Sm amt sanguineous drainage*

Instead of "large bruise," use "2 cm × 3 cm contusion."

General: large bruise

Precise: *2 cm × 3 cm contusion*

Do not use subjective words, such as "good" or "uncooperative," which convey an opinion, imply a judgment, or make an inference. Use objective words that communicate facts or observations. For example, instead of "good night," state objectively what happened during the night to make it a good one for the client: "*OOB to bathroom. Voided 300 mL clear yellow urine.*"

Subjective: good night

Objective: *OOB to bathroom. Voided 300 mL clear yellow urine*

Instead of "ate well," state specifically what the client ate: "*1 egg, 1 piece of toast, juice 120 mL, coffee 240 mL.*"

Subjective: ate well

Objective: *1 egg, 1 piece of toast, juice 120 mL, coffee 240 mL*

Do not write your opinion or interpret data. For example, instead of "was uncooperative," state that the client "*refused medication.*"

Subjective: was uncooperative

Objective: *refused medication*

Instead of "was depressed," state that the client *"was crying."*

Subjective: was depressed

Objective: *was crying*

Subjective data that should be recorded are data that reflect the client's perceptions or experiences. Record such data in the client's own words, e.g., *"I haven't eaten so much in a week"* and use quotation marks. Add the word "stated" or "reports" to show that the words are a direct quote. Do not restate in your own words what the client said, as that could change the client's meaning.

Subjective: Reported: "I haven't eaten so much in a week."

Stated: *"I'm worried about my leg."*

Note that preciseness can sometimes result in longer text.

▶ Activity 2.12: Understanding Precise Wording

Match the precise wording with the corresponding general wording. Write the letter of the precise term in the correct blank. The first one has been done for you.

General	Precise
1. ___f___ bad pain	a. hard firm brown stool
2. ______ dressing in place	b. skin reddened
3. ______ feeling weak	c. 100°F
4. ______ being tired all the time	d. elevated leg 90°
5. ______ eats like a horse	e. without pain
6. ______ warm	f. severe pain (rating of 6–7 on a scale of 0–10), 10 min duration.
7. ______ constipated stool	g. fatigue
8. ______ skin looks red	h. dressing dry and intact
9. ______ does not hurt	i. excellent appetite
10. ______ tap water	j. weakness
11. ______ put leg up on chair	k. 500 mL H_2O

Communication Skills: Blocks to Therapeutic Communication

When used effectively, therapeutic communication helps clients cope with their situation and recover their independence. However, therapeutic communication can also be inadvertently blocked in various ways. Read the dialog between the nurse and Ms. Achu that takes place during the shift. Notice the various ways in which the nurse prevents the effective use of therapeutic communication with the client.

Note: Expressions that are <u>underlined</u> in the dialog are included in Activity 2.2: Understanding Client Talk—Describing Symptoms and Feelings.

Dialog between Nurse and Ms. Achu

Nurse: Good afternoon, Ms. Achu.

Ms. Achu: Hello, nurse. (whispering)

Nurse: How are you feeling?

Ms. Achu: You know, sometimes *I can't seem to catch my breath*. It's really scary having to gasp for air.

Nurse: Well, no wonder. (falling intonation) All those years of smoking have affected your health. (harsh tone of voice)

Ms. Achu: I know, *I wish I had kicked the habit* . . . (staring out the window in deep thought)

Nurse: It's going to be fine; don't worry. But, it's not good to smoke. (rising intonation) You should quit smoking. It causes a lot of health problems.

Ms. Achu: (raising her voice) You're making me feel guilty. (silence)

Nurse: I didn't mean to make you feel that way. It's just the reality of things. . . . (raising her eyebrows) However, we will do the best we can to help you.

Ms. Achu: Well, I just seem to be getting worse since I came to the hospital. I'm having difficulty breathing and *on top of it all* the infection in my urinary tract is not going away. Maybe if you allowed me to take my energy pills, I would be better by now!

Nurse: The UTI should clear up by the time your dose of antibiotics is complete. Herbal supplements are not allowed in the hospital; you've been told that. Sometimes they can cause problems for clients.

Ms. Achu: (silence)

Nurse: Otherwise, is anything else the matter?

Ms. Achu: I just feel useless. I wonder how I will be able to continue working as a tailor… I hope my customers will understand if I need more time to finish alterations. I'm afraid I may lose work and financially . . . *I just don't think I can cope anymore*. (starts sobbing)

Nurse: You'll be fine; you're a strong woman.

Ms. Achu: (silence)

Nurse: Don't you have another source of income? You should ask your family to help you.

Ms. Achu: (silence)

Nurse: Anyway, things will work out; you'll see.

▶ Activity 2.13: Analyzing Effectiveness of Communication

Determine your answers to the following questions about the ineffectiveness of the nurse's communication with Ms. Achu in the dialog.

1. What are some examples of the nurse's ineffective communication with Ms. Achu?

____

____

2. What is the effect of the nurse's ineffective communication on Ms. Achu?

____

____

3. Is the nurse able to address Ms. Achu's concerns? Why or why not?

____

____

4. Do you have any suggestions for how the nurse could be more effective in her communication with Ms. Achu? If so, explain.

____

____

____

____

Expansion of Dialog: Blocks to Therapeutic Communication (Giving Advice, Expressing Disapproval, Judging the Client, and False Reassurance)

Nurses must avoid certain ways of talking that prevent therapeutic communication. Blocks to therapeutic communication do not promote trust and the open communication of feelings.

Giving Advice

Nurses should not give advice or state an opinion about what they think the client should or should not do. Clients may not follow the advice they are given or they may misinterpret the advice or not follow it carefully, and if anything goes wrong, the nurse could be held responsible.

"Should" is commonly used to give advice.

Examples: "You should stop smoking."

"I think you should lose weight."

Rather than give advice, the nurse needs to give clients information or present options and allow clients to make their own decisions and take responsibility for their own choices.

▶ Activity 2.14: Analyzing Dialog for Advice

Look back at the Dialog between Nurse and Ms. Achu. Identify any examples of the nurse giving advice to Ms. Achu. For each example, consider how the advice is given and how the client responds to the advice. What effect does the advice have on Ms. Achu?

____

____

____

____

▶ Activity 2.15: Avoiding Giving Advice

Practice using language that avoids giving advice to the client. Revise the nurse's statements on the left that give advice into statements that encourage the client to consider his or her options. The first one has been done for you.

Nurse's Statement–Gives Advice	Nurse's Statement–Avoids Giving Advice
1. "If you want my opinion, I think you should stop smoking."	1. "Think about your choices. What are the advantages and disadvantages of stopping smoking?"
2. "You ought to try harder."	2. ______________________
3. "The way to discipline your children is to set limits on what they can and cannot do."	3. ______________________
4. "In my opinion, generic drugs are better than brand-name drugs."	4. ______________________
5. "My advice is–go on a diet."	5. ______________________

▶ Activity 2.16: Practice Avoiding Giving Advice

Review the Dialog between Nurse and Ms. Achu. Write down the examples of advice that you identified. What could the nurse have said instead of giving advice? Write alternative statements that the nurse could have used.

Examples of Advice	Alternative Statement
1. ______________________	1. ______________________
2. ______________________	2. ______________________

Expressing Disapproval

Expressing disapproval conveys the message that something is the client's fault. Such a message prevents therapeutic communication and is unlikely to change the client's behavior.

Examples: "You haven't eaten everything on your plate."

"You were told to take your medication 3 times a day."

"Why didn't you call earlier to make an appointment?"

Note the use of "you" statements in these examples. "You" statements often communicate disapproval. If the nurse comes across as expressing disapproval, the client is unlikely to trust the nurse and engage in therapeutic communication. Using "I" statements instead helps to avoid "you" statements.

Note, also, the use of "why" questions in these examples. "Why" questions put clients on the defensive by asking them to explain their feelings or behavior. As a result, the nurse could be perceived as expressing disapproval of a client's feelings or behavior.

There are also ways to communicate disapproval nonverbally, such as through a harsh tone of voice or a falling intonation pattern at the end of a sentence.

▶ Activity 2.17: Analyzing Dialog for Disapproval

Look back at the Dialog between Nurse and Ms. Achu. Identify any examples of the nurse expressing disapproval. For each example, consider how the nurse communicates disapproval and how the client responds to the disapproval. What effect does expressing disapproval have on Ms. Achu?

____

____

____

____

____

▶ Activity 2.18: Avoiding Disapproval

Practice using language that avoids expressing disapproval. Revise the nurse's statements on the left that communicate a message of disapproval into statements that encourage the client to take responsibility for his or her actions. The first one has been done for you.

Nurse's Statement–Expresses Disapproval	Nurse's Statement–Avoids Disapproval
1. "Why did you miss your last 2 appointments?"	1. "I see you missed 2 appointments. Is there something wrong?"
2. "What are you doing out of bed?"	2. ____________________ ____________________ ____________________

3. "You should have seen a doctor about this a long time ago." 3. ____________________

4. "What have you done to yourself?" 4. ____________________

5. "What haven't you touched your food?" 5. ____________________

▶ Activity 2.19: Practice Avoiding Disapproval

Review the Dialog between Nurse and Ms. Achu. Write down the examples of expressing disapproval that you identified. What could the nurse have said instead of expressing disapproval? Write alternative statements that the nurse could have used.

Examples of Disapproval	Alternative Statement
1. ____________________	1. ____________________
2. ____________________	2. ____________________

Judging the Client

The nurse should not judge a client. In judging the client or expressing disapproval, the nurse is likely to intimidate the client, preventing the development of trust in the nurse. "You" statements are frequently used in statements that judge the client, whereas "I" statements are used in nonjudgmental statements.

Positive and Negative Judgment

Although judgment is usually considered to be a negative evaluation, like expressing disapproval, it also refers to positive evaluation. The nurse must avoid both positive and negative evaluation about what is good or bad, right or wrong. If a nurse provides positive evaluation of the client, the client will quickly figure out what the nurse likes to hear and may leave out important health-related information that might cause a negative response by the nurse. Some examples of positive judgment are listed.

Examples: "Your decision to stop smoking was the right one."

"It's good that you're feeling more hopeful about the future."

"You have a very positive attitude."

▸ Activity 2.20: Analyzing Dialog for Judging

Look back at the Dialog between Nurse and Ms. Achu. Identify any examples of the nurse judging the client, both negative and positive judgment. Do your examples of negative judgment overlap with your examples of expressing disapproval? For each example, consider how the nurse communicates judgment and how the client responds to the judgment. What effect does judging have on Ms. Achu?

____

____

____

____

____

▸ Activity 2.21: Avoiding Judging the Client

Practice how to avoid judging the client. Revise the nurse's statements (Judgmental) that communicate a message of judgment. Write statements that practice nonjudgmental communication with clients, to encourage clients to share health-related information. The first one has been done for you.

Repeat the activity, adding nonverbal communication to both the judgmental and nonjudgmental statements. Write out your additions of nonverbal communication. What effect does the nonverbal communication have on both the judgmental and nonjudgmental statements?

Judgmental Statement	Nonjudgmental Statement
1. "You're not taking good care of yourself."	1. It can be difficult learning how to live with a chronic illness.
2. "It's good that you have a lot of friends."	2. ______________________
3. "It's a bad idea to eat sweets in your condition."	3. ______________________
4. "It would be good if you exercised more."	4. ______________________
5. "If you had a more positive attitude, people might like to be around you."	5. ______________________
6. "How can you smoke at your age?"	6. ______________________

▶ Activity 2.22: Practice Avoiding Judging

Review the Dialog between Nurse and Ms. Achu. Write down the examples of judging that you identified. What could the nurse have said instead of judging the client? Write alternative statements that the nurse could have used.

Examples of Judging	Alternative Statement
1. ______________________	1. ______________________
______________________	______________________
2. ______________________	2. ______________________
______________________	______________________

False Reassurance

Nurses sometimes give false reassurance, either by saying something that is not true or by promising something that may not happen. In addition, a nurse can give false reassurance by pretending to comfort a client when the nurse is actually trying to figure out what to do next.

If a client senses that the nurse is giving false reassurance, the client will lose trust in the nurse, and the nurse will not be able to help the client.

Examples: "You have nothing to worry about." (saying something that is not true)

"Don't worry. Everything will be all right." (promising something that may not happen)

"I understand your concern." (as the nurse looks frantically around the room)

Clichés are overused expressions that are often used to give false reassurance.

Examples: "Everything will be all right."

"You don't need to worry."

▶ Activity 2.23: Analyzing Dialog for False Reassurance

Look back at the dialog between the nurse and Ms. Achu. Identify any examples of false reassurance. For each example, consider how the nurse provides false reassurance and how the client responds. What effect does the false reassurance have on Ms. Achu?

____

____

____

____

____

Activity 2.24: Avoiding False Reassurance

Practice how to avoid giving false reassurance to a client. For each statement on the left, decide if the nurse is giving true or false reassurance. If the reassurance is false, decide why it is false. Then, transform it so that the nurse gives reassurance that is true. The first one has been done for you.

Nurse's Statement	Type of Reassurance and Transformation
1. "I hear what you are saying. You are concerned about how your illness will affect your family."	1. True reassurance. No transformation needed.
2. "Don't worry. Everything will work out for the best."	2. ______
3. "Look, it's not so bad. I've seen clients who were much sicker than you get better."	3. ______
4. "It's okay to cry when you feel like it."	4. ______
5. "There's no need to cry. It's not the end of the world, is it?"	5. ______
6. "It will get better soon; you'll see."	6. ______

▶ Activity 2.25: Practice Avoiding False Reassurance

Review the dialog between the nurse and Ms. Achu. Write down the examples of false reassurance that you identified in Activity 2.23. How could the nurse have communicated true reassurance instead? Write alternative statements of true reassurance that the nurse could have used.

Examples of False Reassurance	Statements of True Reassurance
1. ____________________	1. ____________________
2. ____________________	2. ____________________
3. ____________________	3. ____________________
4. ____________________	4. ____________________
5. ____________________	5. ____________________

Culture in Nursing: Cultural Differences in Blocks to Therapeutic Communication (Giving Advice and False Reassurance)

Giving Advice

In some cultures, it is expected that nurses give advice. Clients may expect nurses to give them advice, and nurses may assume it is part of their responsibility to give advice. Instead of giving advice, the nurse needs to give clients information or present options and allow clients to make their own decisions and take responsibility for their own choices.

▶ Activity 2.26: Considering Cultural Differences in Giving Advice

Determine your answers to the following questions.

1. In your culture, are clients ever given advice by health care providers? If so, under what circumstances and why?

2. What is the status of nurses in your culture? Are clients likely to follow the advice or direction of nurses and other health care providers? What are the advantages and disadvantages of this behavior?

3. As a future nurse, would you ever give a client advice? If so, under what circumstances and why?

Giving False Reassurance

In some cultures, it is considered appropriate to comfort clients with false reassurance. However, in the United States it is considered inappropriate, as well as ineffective. Clients may become more anxious, rather than less, especially if the nurse's message differs greatly from the client's perceptions of the problem.

▶ Activity 2.27: Considering Cultural Differences in Giving Reassurance

Determine your answers to the following questions.

1. In your culture, are clients ever given false reassurance? If so, under what circumstances and why?

2. Do you agree with the value in the United States that the client has the right to know his or her prognosis? Why or why not?

3. As a future health care provider, would you ever give a client false reassurance? If so, under what circumstances and why?

Chapter Two Answer Key

Activity 2.1: Considering Complementary and Alternative Medicine

1. Ms. Achu states that she takes herbal supplements "for energy." Besides her stated reason, Ms. Achu may take the supplements because they make her feel better. They may or may not be herbal supplements that are traditional to Ghana, her country of origin, but if they are, they may have been given to her by a traditional healer, someone she trusts and with whom she can communicate easily. She may or may not trust conventional medicine and Western health care providers.

2. Herbals and dietary supplements are widely used in the United States. However, their effectiveness remains largely unproven. In addition, there are concerns about their toxicity and possible side effects, as well as their interactions with other medications. (Source: Comarow, Avery. "Embracing alternative care." US News. Available online. URL: http://www.cbsnews.com/news/embracing-alternative-care/. Posted on February 11, 2009.) It is likely that hospital policy does not allow Ms. Achu to take her herbal supplements while she is in the hospital because they are unsure what is in these supplements. In addition, the staff may be unsure how the supplements might interact with medications that Ms. Achu is receiving while in the hospital. Thus, for her safety, these supplements are being withheld from her. It would be appropriate to allow a client to receive complementary or alternative therapies while in the hospital as long as they do not compromise client safety or interfere with the treatments that the client is already receiving. In many hospitals, clients can request complementary therapies, but some may not be available or permissible. If so, the nurse can suggest alternatives for the client to choose from based on what is offered in the hospital. In addition, nurses can suggest complementary therapies to the client and implement them if the client consents.

3. It is important, regardless of cultural attitudes toward certain behaviors, that a client be treated with dignity and respect. Moreover, it is clear that Ms. Achu would like to quit smoking as she has already tried unsuccessfully to quit several times. The nurse must not judge Ms. Achu or express disapproval for her health issues, nor should the nurse give advice. The nurse needs to provide Ms. Achu with information about smoking and ask if she would like information about new smoking cessation treatment plans.

Activity 2.2: Understanding Client Talk—Describing Symptoms and Feelings

1. The client has difficulty breathing.
2. The client wishes she had stopped smoking (but she did not).
3. The client has an additional problem.
4. The client is having a lot of difficulty managing her problems (and may need help).
5. The client sometimes feels dizzy and lightheaded.
6. The client has a severe headache.
7. The client got worse or became sicker.
8. The client fainted or lost consciousness.

9. __i__ down in the dumps
10. __g__ on top of the world
11. __h__ run down
12. __a__ under the weather
13. __c__ on the mend
14. __b__ out of it
15. __f__ blue
16. __e__ sick to my stomach
17. __d__ like shit

a. not well
b. disconnected, disoriented
c. better, improving, healing
d. terrible
e. nauseous
f. sad
g. very healthy
h. tired, without energy
i. depressed

Medical/Nursing Vocabulary

bronchi: air tubes leading from the trachea into the lungs

chronic obstructive pulmonary disease: disease of the lungs that is characterized by chronic typically irreversible airway obstruction resulting in a slowed rate of exhalation

degenerative joint disease: osteoarthritis typically with onset during middle or old age that is characterized by a progressive loss of joint function, accompanied by pain, swelling, and stiffness

diagnose: to identify a client's condition or illness by examining the client and noting symptoms

dilate: to enlarge, stretch, or cause to expand

exacerbation: worsening of a disease or its symptoms

herbal supplements: substances from plants that have medical properties that are taken to complete or add to a person's treatment

inflammation: the state of being sore, red, and swollen, tender or painful, or having loss of function as a reaction to an infection, irritation, or bodily injury

nasal cannula: a small tube for insertion into the nose, used for administering relatively small amounts of O_2

nicotine patch/nicotine gum: a patch worn on the skin (or gum that is chewed) that contains nicotine, which is absorbed at a constant rate through the skin and into the bloodstream

orthopedic consult: consultation with a doctor specializing in the correction or prevention of deformities, disorders, or injuries of the skeleton and associated structures

passive range of motion (ROM): exercises whereby another person moves each of a client's joints, stretching all muscle groups to the maximum, in order to restore the client's complete range of movement in the joints

primary nurse practitioner: nurse who through advanced training is qualified to assume some of the duties and responsibilities formerly assumed only by a physician, usually nonemergency acute or chronic illness and primary care

pulmonary consult: consultation with a doctor specializing in the lungs

pulse oximeter: instrument that measures continuously the degree of oxygen saturation of the circulating blood

semi-Fowler's position: HOB is raised at a 30°–45° angle while the client is lying supine or on the back to promote lung expansion and relief from lying down (In Fowler's position, HOB is at 45°–60° angle; in high Fowler's position, HOB is at 80°–90°; and in low Fowler's position, HOB is 15°–30°.)

sodium: chemical element that is the basic substance in salt

sputum: mucus which is formed in the inflamed nose, throat, or lungs, especially the lungs and bronchi in diseased states, and is coughed up; may also contain pus and blood

urinary tract infection: infection in the tract through which urine passes, which consists of the renal tubules and renal pelvis of the kidney, the ureters, the bladder, and the urethra

urine culture and sensitivity: lab test that checks if bacteria are present in the urine and determines which antimicrobials will be effective

vitals: short for vital signs, or the signs of life: specifically, the pulse rate, respiration rate, body temperature, blood pressure, and oxygen saturation of a person

▶ Activity 2.3: Route of Administration

1. ___po___ by mouth
2. ___subcut___ subcutaneous
3. ___ID___ intradermal
4. ___IM___ intramuscular
5. ___IV___ intravenous
6. ___gtt___ drop
7. ___MDI___ metered dose inhaler
8. ___R___ rectally

▶ Activity 2.4: Identifying Medication Orders, Labs, Tests, and Nursing Actions in Scenario #2

Medications

Oxygen	Increases oxygen blood level; 2 L via nasal cannula
Albuterol	Dilates bronchial tubes (to increase air flow to lungs); 2 puffs BID
Normal saline	Maintains hydration and fluid balance; 0.9% IV running at 75 mL/hr
Acetaminophen	Relieves pain; 325–650 mg PO PRN
Lisinopril	Stabilizes high blood pressure; 20 mg PO daily
Prednisone	Reduces inflammation (to reduce symptoms of DJD and COPD); 10 mg PO BID
Gentamicin	Fights infection; 70 mg IVPB q8h

The additional information that is provided is: amount of medication, route of medication, and frequency of administration, in that order.

Labs/Tests

CBC lab

urine culture and sensitivity

Nursing Actions*

monitor O_2 sats

elevate HOB at least 30° in semi-Fowler's position

take vitals every 8 hours

perform passive ROM

maintain on low sodium diet

perform focused respiratory assessment

perform focused musculoskeletal assessment

*Note that consults are not included here, as they are not performed by a nurse or nursing assistive personnel (NAP).

▶ Activity 2.5: Plan of Care: Planning for Client's Care

1. Exacerbation of COPD (chronic obstructive pulmonary disease) and UTI (urinary tract infection)
2. DJD (degenerative joint disease), HTN (hypertension), and COPD
3. BID (twice daily), at 8:00 a.m. and 8:00 p.m.
4. NS (normal saline) and gentamicin
5. VS q8h, continuous O_2 sat monitoring, focused respiratory, focused musculoskeletal

Nursing Diagnosis: Planning Holistic Care for Ms. Achu

The intervention "Nurse will offer hand massage to enhance relaxation and decrease anxiety by the end of shift" reflects care of Ms. Achu's psychosocial need to reduce her anxiety.

▶ Activity 2.6: Nursing Diagnosis: Nursing Interventions and Desired Outcomes

Nursing Intervention	Desired Outcome
1. ___d___ Nurse will teach client huff coughing technique by the end of shift.	a. Client will report less fatigue from breathing by the end of shift.
2. ___b___ Nurse will keep head of bed elevated above 30 degrees, encourage use of inspiratory spirometer, and assess client's breathing and oxygen saturation throughout shift.	b. O_2 saturation will improve to 90% by the end of shift.
3. ___a___ Nurse will administer inhaler medications as ordered and provide mouth care after inhalers during shift.	c. Client will report less anxiety by the end of shift.
4. ___c___ Nurse will offer hand massage to enhance relaxation and decrease anxiety by the end of shift.	d. Client will have decreased crackles heard over lung fields within an hour of treatment.

Activity 2.7: Understanding Qualifiers

Qualifiers

compromised	disabled	impaired
decreased	disturbed	ineffective
deficient	dysfunctional	interrupted
delayed	imbalanced	perceived

Definitions

1. disabled — limited or unable
2. deficient — not sufficient in degree, amount, or quality
3. interrupted — to break the continuity of a process
4. imbalanced — out of balance or proportion
5. perceived — to become aware of through use of the senses
6. compromised — made vulnerable to threat of infection or injury
7. ineffective — not producing the desired or intended effect
8. delayed — slow, late, or postponed
9. disturbed — agitated; interrupted
10. dysfunctional — functioning that is abnormal
11. decreased — smaller in degree, size, or amount
12. impaired — weakened, damaged, reduced

Activity 2.8: Identifying Qualifiers in Diagnostic Statements

Qualifiers

Impaired

Activity 2.9: Understanding Telephone Order Report

1. NS
2. Formoterol, beclomethasone, metaxalone, Lasix
3. 800 mg; now and in 6 hours
4. To prevent fluid accumulation in her lungs and possible pneumonia
5. HOB is elevated to 45° in telephone order compared to 30° in the scenario because of the worsening of the client's condition. HOB is higher now to decrease pressure in the chest and ease the work of breathing.
6. 4 L of O_2 are ordered in the telephone order compared to 2 L in the scenario because the client is in is SOB and has distressed breathing. More oxygen is needed to provide relief.

▶ Activity 2.10: Providing Holistic Care

1. The client's anxiety secondary to her shortness of breath is identified as one of the problems in the progress note. In addition, a reduction in the client's anxiety is listed as one of the desired outcomes in the care of the client. Specific ways to address the client's anxiety in the plan of care include encouraging client to use incentive spirometer; teaching client importance of smoking cessation; and providing a quiet, healing environment, music therapy, and hand massage to promote client's well-being. The client is also encouraged to inform the nurse about any concerns she has regarding her health and care. In addition, the client's health status and progress continue to be monitored and medications administered per MAR, and passive ROM continues to be performed. In sum, the client's anxiety is addressed at both the psychosocial and physiological levels. In addition, the family and the client's primary care provider are included in a discussion about the client's plan of care, reflecting a holistic perspective of the client as member of a family system and as part of a larger network of support and care.

2. In addition to providing a quiet healing environment, the nurse provides two complementary therapies to promote the client's well-being: music therapy and hand massage.

▶ Activity 2.11: Understanding Medical/Nursing Terminology

Medical/Nursing Terminology

a. palpitations
b. anorectic
c. radiate
d. intermittent pain
e. serous drainage
f. abduct
g. diaphoretic
h. voided
i. tingling
j. edema
k. sanguineous drainage
l. substernal
m. flex
n. brown fluid
o. copious
p. epistaxis
q. clear fluid
r. dyspneic
s. expels flatus
t. at rest
u. has full ROM
v. marked pallor
w. wet pack
x. emesis

Layperson's Terms

1. ___h___ went to the bathroom
2. ___f___ move
3. ___m___ bend
4. ___l___ under the breast
5. ___c___ spread out
6. ___g___ sweating
7. ___i___ pins and needles
8. ___a___ abnormally rapid or irregular heart beat
9. ___b___ no appetite
10. ___e___ yellowish liquid (from wound)

11. ____k____ bloody liquid (from wound)
12. ____d____ pain that comes and goes
13. ____j____ swelling
14. ____v____ very pale
15. ____r____ has difficulty breathing
16. ____t____ when resting
17. ____w____ wet towel
18. ____u____ is able to move wrist
19. ____p____ bloody nose
20. ____x____ vomiting
21. ____s____ passes a lot of gas
22. ____q____ water-like liquid
23. ____n____ brownish liquid
24. ____o____ large amount

▶ Activity 2.12: Understanding Precise Wording

General		Precise
1. ____f____	bad pain	a. hard firm brown stool
2. ____h____	dressing in place	b. skin reddened
3. ____j____	feeling weak	c. 100°F
4. ____g____	being tired all the time	d. elevated leg 90°
5. ____i____	eats like a horse	e. without pain
6. ____c____	warm	f. severe pain (rating of 7–9 on a scale of 0–10), 10 min duration.
7. ____a____	constipated stool	g. fatigue
8. ____b____	skin looks red	h. dressing dry and intact
9. ____e____	does not hurt	i. excellent appetite
10. ____k____	tap water	j. weakness
11. ____d____	put leg up on chair	k. 500 mL H_2O

▶ Activity 2.13: Analyzing Effectiveness of Communication

1. Answers will vary, but students should notice the negative comments that the nurse makes. For example, in response to Ms. Achu's complaint that "it's really scary having to gasp for air," the nurse says: "Well, no wonder... All those years of smoking have affected your health." The nurse also seems to belittle Ms. Achu's concerns about her health and the effect of her health on her work by her overuse of clichés, for example, "It's going to be fine; don't worry" and "Things will come together; you'll see."

2. Ms. Achu is silenced multiple times because of the nurse's negative comments. For example, after the nurse says: "Well, no wonder... All those years of smoking have affected your health," Ms. Achu responds with regret but her voice trails off, as she looks out the window lost in her thoughts. After the nurse's second negative comment, "It's not good to smoke," and her advice, "You should quit smoking," Ms. Achu responds defensively. She raises her voice and says, "You're making me feel guilty," and is then silent. The nurse is unsympathetic to Ms. Achu's complaint that she is not able to take her energy pills, and the nurse also does not acknowledge when Ms. Achu begins sobbing. The nurse's untherapeutic response both times results in complete silence from Ms. Achu.

3. Clearly, the nurse is not able to address Ms. Achu's concerns. She has not allowed Ms. Achu the opportunity to talk about her fears of not being able to breathe easily or her concerns about how her health will affect her work.

4. Answers will vary, but essentially the nurse needs to listen to Ms. Achu without passing judgment or expressing disapproval for her past actions. She needs to stop using clichés and show true empathy and concern for the client.

▶ Activity 2.14: Analyzing Dialog for Advice

The nurse gives advice twice to Ms. Achu. The first time, the nurse states, "You should quit smoking." The second time, the nurse states: "You should ask your family to help you." In response to the first advice, Ms. Achu gets defensive and raises her voice, saying, "You're making me feel guilty." After the second advice, Ms. Achu does not respond at all. In both instances, the advice is given using the verb "should," and in both cases, the advice prevents the effective use of therapeutic communication.

▶ Activity 2.15: Avoiding Giving Advice

Nurse's Statement—Gives Advice	Nurse's Statement—Avoids Giving Advice
1. "If you want my opinion, I think you should stop smoking."	1. "Think about your choices. What are the advantages and disadvantages of quitting smoking?"
2. "You ought to try harder."	2. "What is holding you back, do you think?"
3. "The way to discipline your child is to set limits on what they can and cannot do."	3. "What are some ways you could try to discipline your child?"
4. "In my opinion, generic drugs are better than brand-name drugs."	4. "Do you know the difference between generic and brand-name drugs?"
5. "My advice is—go on a diet."	5. "How can you lose the weight you need to?"

Activity 2.16: Practice Avoiding Giving Advice

Examples of Advice	Alternative Statement
1. "You should quit smoking."	1. "Would you like to try and quit smoking again? There is a new medication for people who have had difficulty quitting. If you like, I can get you some information about it and you can talk with the doctor when he comes to see you."
2. "You should ask your family to help you."	2. "Are there people you know who could help out?"

Activity 2.17: Analyzing Dialog for Disapproval

The nurse expresses disapproval at least twice to Ms. Achu. The first time, in response to Ms. Achu's complaint that "it's really scary having to gasp for air," the nurse says: "Well, no wonder… All those years of smoking have affected your health." This comment essentially blames Ms. Achu for her difficulty breathing, a comment that causes Ms. Achu to become sad. Later in the interview after Ms. Achu expresses concern about the effect of her health on her ability to work, the nurse asks: "Don't you have another source of income?" suggesting that Ms. Achu is to blame if she does not. Ms. Achu does not respond. Clearly, the nurse's expression of disapproval prevents the use of therapeutic communication with the client.

Activity 2.18: Avoiding Disapproval

Nurse's Statement–Expresses Disapproval	Nurse's Statement–Avoids Disapproval
1. "Why did you miss your last 2 appointments?"	1. "I see you missed 2 appointments. Is there something wrong?"
2. "What are you doing out of bed?"	2. "I see you're out of bed. Is there a problem I can help you with?"
3. "You should have seen a doctor about this a long time ago."	3. "This looks serious. It should be checked by a doctor immediately."
4. "What have you done to yourself?"	4. "Can you tell me what happened?"
5. "Why haven't you touched your food?"	5. "I notice you haven't eaten anything. How are you feeling?"

Activity 2.19: Practice Avoiding Disapproval

Examples of Disapproval	Alternative Statement
1. "Well, no wonder… All those years of smoking have affected your health."	1. "Tell me more about your concerns."
2. "Don't you have another source of income?"	2. "It must be hard not being able to work right now."

Activity 2.20: Analyzing Dialog for Judging

The nurse tells Ms. Achu, "It's not good to smoke." Although the focus is on smoking, it's clear that negative judgment of Ms. Achu is implied for smoking. Ms. Achu responds by getting defensive, saying, "You're making me feel guilty," followed by silence. Feeling judged, Ms. Achu does not open up and talk about her concerns about her health, as she started to at the beginning of the dialog. Toward the end of the dialog, the nurse states, "You're a strong woman." By judging Ms. Achu positively for being strong, the nurse may have created a block to therapeutic communication, as Ms. Achu may be less likely to open up in the future if what she has to say could imply that she is not strong.

Activity 2.21: Avoiding Judging the Client

Judgmental Statements	Nonjudgmental Statements
1. "You're not taking good care of yourself."	1. "It can be difficult learning how to live with a chronic illness."
2. "It's good that you have a lot of friends."	2. "Do you know people you can count on?"
3. "It's a bad idea to eat sweets in your condition."	3. "I'd like to talk with you about your diet."
4. "It would be good if you exercised more."	4. "What are the benefits of exercise?"
5. "If you had a more positive attitude, people might like to be around you."	5. "How does your attitude affect others?"
6. "How can you smoke at your age?"	6. "What are some reasons to stop smoking?"

Activity 2.22: Practice Avoiding Judging

Examples of Judging	Alternative Statement
1. "It's not good to smoke."	1. "Let's focus on what we can do now to improve your health."
2. "You're a strong woman."	2. "It's okay to cry."

Activity 2.23: Analyzing Dialog for False Reassurance

There are numerous instances of false reassurance in the dialog, particularly through the use of clichés: The nurse says, "It's going to be fine; don't worry," after Ms. Achu expresses regret for having smoked, though she is unable to finish her sentence. By using a cliché here, the nurse avoids having to respond to Ms. Achu's expression of her feelings. After Ms. Achu says, "You're making me feel guilty," the nurse responds defensively herself, saying "I didn't mean to make you feel that way," followed by more clichés:"It's just the reality of things" and "We will do the best we can to help you." Toward the end of the dialog, when Ms. Achu begins to cry, the nurse responds once more with clichés: "You'll be fine" and "Things will work out, you'll see." By using clichés, the nurse shows that she has not listened to Ms. Achu's concerns and is more concerned about her own discomfort than helping Ms. Achu to work through her fears and concerns through the effective use of therapeutic communication.

▶ Activity 2.24: Avoiding False Reassurance

Nurse's Statement	Type of Reassurance and Transformation
1. "I hear what you are saying. You are concerned about how your illness will affect your family."	1. True reassurance. No transformation needed.
2. "Don't worry. Everything will work out for the best."	2. False reassurance. **Transformation:** "You seem worried. Is there anything I can do?"
3. "Look, it's not so bad. I've seen clients who were in worse shape than you who have gotten better."	3. False reassurance. **Transformation:** "This hospital specializes in treating clients with your condition. We have the most experienced doctors at this hospital and the latest equipment to treat your condition."
4. "It's okay to cry when you feel like it."	4. True reassurance. No transformation needed.
5. "There's no need to cry. It's not the end of the world, is it?"	5. False reassurance. **Transformation:** "It's okay to cry. I can wait for you."
6. "It will get better soon; you'll see."	6. False reassurance. **Transformation:** "I know you're concerned that your progress is slow, but it will take time to fully recover the use of your arm."

▶ Activity 2.25: Practice Avoiding False Reassurance

Examples of False Reassurance	Statements of True Reassurance
1. "It's going to be fine; don't worry."	1. "It's okay to feel sad."
2. "It's just the reality of things."	2. "Smoking does make the COPD worse."
3. "We will do the best we can to help you."	3. "I will do everything I can to make you comfortable during your stay."
4. "You'll be fine."	4. "Would you like me to contact the social worker to talk with you about any services that might be available for you while you recover your strength?"
5. "Things will come together; you'll see."	5. "With rest, the right medication, and a smoke-free environment, you will feel better."

▶ Activity 2.26: Considering Cultural Differences in Giving Advice

1. In some cultures, nurses (and doctors) are expected to give advice.
2. Answers will vary. Clients do not automatically follow the advice they are given by health care providers. Instead of giving advice, the nurse should give clients information or present options and allow clients to make their own decisions and take responsibility for their own choices. If advice is given, clients could misinterpret it or not follow it carefully, and if anything goes wrong, the nurse could be held responsible.
3. Answers will vary, but in general, nurses should not give a client advice.

▶ Activity 2.27: Considering Cultural Differences in Giving Reassurance

1. In some cultures, clients are given false reassurance to comfort them and ease their suffering, especially in the case of a terminal illness.

2. Answers will vary.

3. Answers will vary, but in the case of a terminal illness, if the family has decided not to tell the client and the client has willingly turned over the authority to make decisions to the family, it may be appropriate not to say something that could undermine the family's plan.

Providing Culturally Competent Care

3

Learning Objectives

- Providing culturally competent care
- Understanding language clients use to describe symptoms and feelings
- Learning medical/nursing abbreviations related to medication orders: Frequency of administration
- Identifying medication orders, labs, tests, and nursing actions
- Understanding the language of nursing diagnoses: Etiology and signs and symptoms
- Documenting client care: Using medical/nursing abbreviations, acronyms, and concise wording
- Taking a pain history
- Understanding language clients use to rate and describe pain
- Understanding and using interviewing skills effectively: Open-ended questions, focused questions, probes, paraphrases, requests for clarification, discrepancy tests, summaries, and closure
- Recognizing cultural differences in pain management

Scenario #3

Client: Hmong male, 64 yo

Diagnosis: Angina

History: Myocardial infarction, hypertension, atherosclerosis, hypercholesterolemia

Mr. Dan Yang is a 64-year-old Hmong man diagnosed with **angina** who was admitted to the **cardiac/telemetry** unit. He came in **complaining** of **intense** chest pain during the night. He stated that he felt a tightness in his chest, like an elephant sitting on him. He also stated that the pain increases with **exertion**. He rated his chest pain at 8 on a scale of 0 to 10. The pain was **radiating** to his shoulders, arms, and upper abdomen. He is sometimes SOB (short of breath); at work yesterday he had to take several rest breaks. He stated that **over-the-counter analgesics** do not relieve the **acute** pain, so **pain management** has been quite challenging. He has **diaphoresis** and feels weak. He has **tachycardia** and JVD (**jugular venous distension**). Upon doing a **health history** during **triage**, the admitting nurse found that pt had an MI (**myocardial infarction**) 4 years ago. **Cardiac catheterization** was done at that time. Pt also has HTN (hypertension), **atherosclerosis**, and **hypercholesterolemia**. He is Full Code. He has NKA (no known allergies) and is on **bed rest**. The attending physician ordered a nitroglycerin 0.5 mg tablet stat to decrease **myocardial** oxygen demand, a **chewable** aspirin 325 mg once to decrease **platelet** activity and clot formation, and hydromorphone (Dilaudid)1.5 mg IV push PRN q3–4hr to relieve pain. The physician ordered O_2 at 2L via NC to increase oxygenation if O_2 sats fall below 90%. Mr. Yang also has orders for **electrolyte** labs, **troponin** lab, CBC lab, and **stress test**. His vitals should be checked q15 min until there is chest pain relief. His diet status is NPO at this time. Pt also needs focused cardiac and respiratory assessments. The physician put in a **cardiology consult** for further assessment and a **dietician consult** related to high cholesterol levels. Mr. Yang runs a restaurant that he co-owns with his brother. Before Mr. Yang came to the hospital, he was given traditional treatments. The bruises on his chest are the result of cupping[†] and prick marks on his fingers from pricking of skin[§] to release pressure. His wife and 3 grandchildren (ages 4, 6, and 12 years) have been with him since admission. His wife speaks little English, so a Hmong interpreter is needed during consultations and updates. Through an interpreter, the wife said that a shaman[*f*] is on his way to see Mr. Yang. Mr. Yang's condition has not improved since the traditional treatments, so a soul-calling ceremony[¶] is being planned.

[†] *Cupping* is a procedure used to release the buildup of pressure in the body, which is thought to be the cause of chest pain and other ailments. A glass cup is placed on the site of pain and then heated to create a vacuum. The procedure causes a bruise, which is sometimes misinterpreted as physical abuse by health care providers.

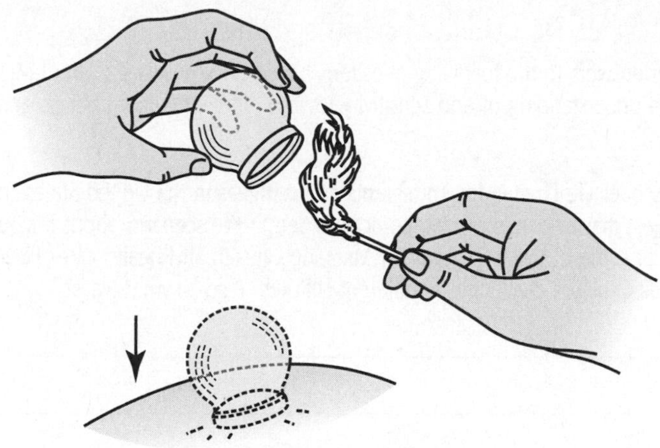

Figure 3-1: Cupping

§Pricking of the skin is done with a needle, often in conjunction with cupping, at the site of the bruised skin. The procedure is thought to release pressure and toxins that cause the chest pain. The blood is then examined. If the blood is dark and thick, the illness is thought to be serious.

ƒA shaman is an intermediary between this world and the spirit world. A shaman performs a ritual ceremony during which he or she enters the spirit world in search of the lost soul.

¶A serious health issue is sometimes interpreted in traditional Hmong culture as a loss of soul. Therefore, a shaman is called in to perform a soul-calling ceremony.

Critical Thinking Skills: Providing Culturally Competent Care

Nurses need to be aware of and sensitive to beliefs and practices around health and health care that may be different from their own, while not making assumptions or stereotyping someone based on that person's cultural or ethnic background.

Being culturally competent is part of thinking critically and providing holistic care to clients. Nurses need to listen to clients to find out what they believe about health and illness and to understand culturally influenced health behaviors. Cultural competence requires nurses to consider a client's cultural as well as psychosocial and spiritual needs. Providing culturally competent care improves the quality of care and health outcomes for clients from culturally and linguistically diverse backgrounds.

▶ Activity 3.1: Considering Traditional Beliefs and Practices

Determine your answers to the following questions based on Scenario #3 about Mr. Yang. How would you incorporate understanding of and sensitivity toward different cultural beliefs and practices in your care of the client?

1. In what ways does life change for immigrants and refugees in the United States (or another country of migration)? What evidence of change do you see in the scenario about Mr. Yang? What are the implications of some of these changes for Mr. Yang's health and health care? Have you experienced different kinds of health challenges in different cultures? If so, in what ways?

____

____

____

____

____

2. Why is a shaman on the way to the hospital? How should the hospital and health care staff at the hospital respond to the shaman in Mr. Yang's room and to the soul-calling ceremony that is being planned? How should the health care team respond to the traditional treatments that Mr. Yang has already received? Are there certain beliefs and practices that are important to you in maintaining your health and in receiving health care that are not practiced in U.S. health care?

____

____

____

____

____

3. What is or should be the responsibility of hospitals to provide interpreters for clients and family members who are not fluent in English? Is it appropriate for children of clients to serve as interpreters? Why or why not? Have you or your family members experienced challenges with the health care system in the United States (or another country of migration) because of language differences? If so, in what ways?

____

____

____

____

____

Understanding and Using Language Effectively in Health Care Settings

The language used in health care settings is different from general, conversational English. Nurses must use medical/nursing terminology as well as specialized ways of communicating with clients. In addition, nurses must understand the language that clients use in the health care setting.

Client Talk: Describing Symptoms and Feelings

Clients use a variety of words and expressions to describe how they are feeling. Many of these words and expressions are colloquial and idiomatic. You may not find them in a standard English dictionary and they cannot be understood word for word. Keep a list of expressions you hear that you do not understand and ask a friend or colleague who is a native English speaker or an experienced nurse what the expressions mean. To communicate effectively with clients and colleagues, you need to understand spoken, idiomatic English. With time, you may even start to use the same words and expressions.

▶ Activity 3.2: Understanding Client Talk—Describing Symptoms and Feelings

What do the following expressions spoken by Mr. Yang in the Dialog between Nurse and Mr. Yang later in this chapter mean? Write down your understanding of each expression.

1. "The pain was killing me." ____________________
2. "I will become dependent on painkillers." ____________________
3. "What if I don't make it?" ____________________

What do the following additional expressions mean? Write down your understanding of each expression.

4. "I caught a nasty bug." ____________________
5. "I've lost my appetite." ____________________
6. "My stomach has been giving me a hard time." ____________________
7. "I can't keep anything down." ____________________
8. "I'm bringing up blood." ____________________

Match the definition with each expression or idiom. Write the letter of the definition in the correct blank.

Idiom	Definition
11. ________ black out	a. become sick with an illness
12. ________ break out	b. restore to consciousness
13. ________ bring to	c. recover from a serious illness
14. ________ come down with	d. lose consciousness, faint
15. ________ pull through	e. show a rash or other skin disorder

Medical/Nursing Vocabulary

How many of the bolded medical/nursing words used in Scenario #3 about Mr. Yang do you already know? For those words you do not know, look them up in a nursing textbook, an English language medical dictionary, or online resources. Refer to the definitions in the Answer Key for Chapter Three, as needed.

Expansion of Scenario #3: Responses to Pain

Nurses need to assess clients for signs that they are experiencing pain, as some clients may choose not to talk about their pain or choose to downplay it. If nurses do not accurately assess a client's experience of pain, they may not provide adequate pain medication.

Upon admission to the hospital, Mr. Yang exhibits various physiological and behavioral responses to pain. Later in the interview with the nurse, he exhibits other responses to pain.

▶ Activity 3.3: Identifying Responses to Pain

Review Scenario #3 and write Mr. Yang's physiologic and behavioral responses to pain. After you have read the Dialog between Nurse and Mr. Yang later in this chapter, add any additional responses to pain that he exhibits. Categorize the responses as either physiologic or behavioral.

____

____

____

____

____

Finally, use a nursing textbook or online resources to add at least 3–4 additional responses to pain. Categorize the responses as either physiologic or behavioral.

Physiologic Responses to Pain

1. ____
2. ____
3. ____
4. ____

Behavioral Responses to Pain

1. ____
2. ____
3. ____
4. ____

Medical/Nursing Abbreviations

Identify as many of the abbreviations from Scenario #3 about Mr. Yang as you can. Refer, as needed, to the list of Medical/Nursing Abbreviations in the Appendix.

Expansion of Medical/Nursing Abbreviations: Medication Orders (Frequency of Administration)

The medications that Mr. Yang is currently taking are included in Scenario #3. Abbreviations and acronyms are commonly used in medication orders.

Medication Orders

There are 7 parts to a medication order. (See the Medication Orders section in Chapter One to review the 7 parts.) Chapter One talked about dose (part 4), and Chapter Two discussed route of administration (part 5). Frequency of administration is the sixth part.

▶ Activity 3.4: Frequency of Administration

Write the correct abbreviation in the blank for each word or phrase used in medication orders. The first one has been done for you.

× # AC am BID $\bar{c}$ hr/h HS PC PRN

pm q2h q4h q6h qh qhs QID $\bar{s}$ stat TID

1. ___stat___ at once, immediately
2. __________ as needed
3. __________ morning
4. __________ afternoon
5. __________ number
6. __________ times
7. __________ twice a day
8. __________ 3 times a day
9. __________ 4 times a day
10. __________ hour
11. __________ every hour
12. __________ every 2 hours
13. __________ every 4 hours
14. __________ every 6 hours
15. __________ at bedtime

16. __________ every night at bedtime

17. __________ before meals

18. __________ after meals

19. __________ with

20. __________ without

Expansion of Scenario #3: Understanding Medication Orders, Labs, Tests, and Nursing Actions

When Mr. Yang is admitted to the hospital, he is assessed by the attending physician, who orders medications, labs (laboratory tests), and other tests for him. In addition, both the physician and the nurse who is assigned to care for Mr. Yang on the medical-surgical unit determine appropriate nursing actions. Some of these nursing care actions are carried out by the nurse; some are carried out by licensed practical or vocational nurses (LPNs/LVNs) or nursing assistive personnel (NAP); and some are carried out by other health care professionals.

▶ Activity 3.5: Identifying Medication Orders, Labs, Tests, and Nursing Actions in Scenario #3

Write down the medications that are ordered for Mr. Yang. Why is each medication ordered? What information is provided for each medication, and in what order? For each medication, write the information that is provided.

Medications

____

____

____

____

____

Write down the labs and other tests that have been ordered and the nursing actions that have been planned for Mr. Yang.

Labs/Tests

____

____

____

____

____

Nursing Actions

____

____

____

____

____

Expansion of Scenario #3: Plan of Care

When nursing students prepare for clinical, they often use forms like the Plan of Care (Figure 3-2) to record essential information about the client from the client's record and to plan for the client's care. Note that the route of medication is not always specified on the plan of care, as nurses would refer to the Medical Administration Record (MAR) before administering medications. This Plan of Care reflects care for Mr. Yang during the day shift thc day after Mr. Yang was admitted to the hospital. The vital signs recorded were taken at the beginning of the shift.

Figure 3-2: Plan of Care
Scenario #3

ROOM
1758

DIET
NPO

OTHER
Full Code

Nitroglycerin 0.5 mg sublingual tablet (stat)

T	P	RR	BP
98.9	84	17	140/95

O_2 sats 94% RA*

INITIALS
NJ

ACTIVITY
Bed rest

NOTES
Pt sometimes SOB

Dx
Angina

IVs
Hydromorphone 1.5 mg IV push PRN q3–4hr

MHx
MI

HTN

Atherosclerosis

Hypercholesterolemia

LABS/TESTS/APPTS
Electrolytes

Troponin

CBC

Stress test

Cardiology consult

Dietician consult

ASSESSMENTS
VS q15min until decrease in chest pain

Focused cardiac

Focused respiratory

MDs
Dr. Suki

TREATMENTS
O_2 at 2 L via NC if O_2 sats fall below 90%

ALLERGY
NKA

PAIN
8/10 chest pain

OUTPUTS
N/A

0700/1900	0800/2000	0900/2100	1000/2200	1100/1300	1200/2400
Chewable aspirin 325 mg (once)					
1300/0100	**1400/0200**	**1500/0300**	**1600/0400**	**1700/0500**	**1800/0600**

*RA (room air) = regular conditions of breathing, without any added oxygen

▶ Activity 3.6: Plan of Care: Planning for Client's Care

Answer the following questions with information that is provided in the Plan of Care regarding Mr. Yang.

1. What is Mr. Yang's diagnosis?

____

____

2. What is Mr. Yang's medical history?

____

____

3. How much hydromorphone (Dilaudid) is Mr. Yang given and how often?

____

____

4. How often should the nurse check Mr. Yang's vitals?

____

____

5. What assessments are planned for Mr. Yang?

____

____

Nursing Diagnosis: Planning Culturally Competent Care for Mr. Yang

Based on the information provided in the client's record and the nurse's assessment* of the client, the nurse writes a nursing diagnosis and a goal for treating the client. The nurse also identifies nursing interventions and desired outcomes to accomplish that goal. In planning holistic care for Mr. Yang, the nurse plans interventions that address Mr. Yang's psychosocial and cultural needs, as well as his physiologic needs. Review the interventions in Activity 3.7. Which nursing intervention is responsive to Mr. Yang's cultural values and beliefs regarding health care?

*A physical assessment is usually conducted when a client is first admitted to the hospital, either a head-to-toe assessment or a focused assessment on a specific problem area, followed by a head-to-toe assessment, as needed. Information from this assessment is included in the client's record and is reviewed by the nurse caring for Mr. Yang.

Nursing Diagnosis: Acute pain related to decreased myocardial blood flow and decreased oxygen supply as manifested by shortness of breath, tachycardia, and client stating: "I have tightness in my chest and feel weak."

Goal: Client will report decrease in chest pain.

▶ Activity 3.7: Nursing Diagnosis: Nursing Interventions and Desired Outcomes

Match each Desired Outcome for Mr. Yang with the corresponding Nursing Intervention.

Write the letter of the Desired Outcome in the correct blank.

Nursing Intervention	Desired Outcome
1. __________ Nurse will administer oxygen, as ordered by physician, throughout shift.	a. Client will report decreased anxiety by the end of shift.
2. __________ Nurse will assess pain, both using the pain rating scale and assessing for signs and symptoms, and administer pain medication as needed throughout shift.	b. Client will maintain oxygen saturation level of greater than 90% throughout shift.
3. __________ Nurse will assess vital signs every 15 minutes throughout shift until there is a decrease in chest pain.	c. Client will report pain level of 3 (scale 0–10) within 1 hour of analgesic administration.
4. __________ Nurse will encourage client to express any concerns and ask questions about treatment and procedures, and will welcome participation of family members in such discussions by the end of shift.	d. Client will maintain stable vital signs throughout shift: blood pressure (120/80), pulse (60–100), respiration rate (12–20), temperature (98.6°), and O_2 sats (95–100%).

Expansion of Nursing Diagnosis: Understanding the Language of Nursing Diagnoses (Etiology and Signs and Symptoms)

Most nursing diagnoses consist of 3 parts:

1. Problem (P): Statement of the client's response to the illness or condition
2. Etiology (E): Factors that contribute to or probable causes of the client's response
3. Signs and Symptoms (S): Defining characteristics, or cluster of signs and symptoms, as manifested by the client that indicate the problem category

In Chapter Two, you were introduced to the Problem, the first part of the nursing diagnosis.

Etiology (E)

The second part of the nursing diagnosis states the Etiology of the Problem—that is, the likely causes or contributing factors to the client's response to the illness. Several causes are usually listed, as in the following example:

Problem	Constipation
Etiology	Prolonged laxative use, decreased oral fluids, decreased dietary fiber

Signs and Symptoms (S/S)

The third part of the nursing diagnosis states the Signs and Symptoms, or the defining characteristics of the Problem that the client exhibits. The symptoms are the subjective data that the client has experienced, and the signs are the objective data that the nurse observes. The nurse uses these signs and symptoms to select the appropriate Problem.

In this example, the Signs and Symptoms are those defining characteristics of constipation that the client has experienced:

Problem	Constipation
Signs and Symptoms	abdominal pain, feeling of rectal fullness, severe flatus, unable to pass stool

<u>**Note:**</u> Risk diagnoses consist of the Problem and Etiology only; Signs and Symptoms are not included for a condition that does not yet exist. Likewise, health promotion diagnoses consist only of the diagnosis. There is no Etiology for a condition that is healthy.

Connectors/Qualifiers Used in Nursing Diagnoses

Specific words are used to connect or modify parts of the nursing diagnosis. The Problem and Etiology are linked using the words *related to*, suggesting probable causation based on observation of the client's signs and symptoms. *Related to* is often abbreviated as R/T, as in the following example:

Problem and Etiology	Constipation related to prolonged laxative use → Constipation R/T prolonged laxative use

When the Problem requires more data, the word *possible* is used. When the Etiology requires more data, *possibly* is used, as in the following examples:

Problem	Possible situational low self-esteem R/T loss of job and rejection by family
Etiology	Disturbed thought processes possibly R/T unfamiliar surroundings

Information about the illness or medical diagnosis is included in the Etiology following *secondary to,* as shown in the following example:

Etiology	Risk for impaired skin integrity R/T decreased peripheral circulation secondary to diabetes

The Etiology and Signs and Symptoms are linked using the words *as evidenced by* or *as manifested by*, often abbreviated as a.m.b., as in the following example:

Etiology and Signs and Symptoms	Constipation R/T prolonged laxative use a.m.b. abdominal pain, feeling of rectal fullness, severe flatus, unable to pass stool

▶ Activity 3.8: Understanding Problems and Etiologies

Match each probable cause or Etiology with the corresponding Problem. Write the letter of the Etiology in the correct blank.

Problem		Etiology
1. __________	Ineffective breastfeeding	a. R/T disruption of family routine secondary to hospitalization
2. __________	Impaired physical mobility	b. R/T unrelenting care requirements and physical disabilities secondary to stroke
3. __________	Impaired verbal communication	c. R/T to knowledge deficit: nonpharmacological pain management
4. __________	Disturbed body image	d. R/T increased dependency secondary to trauma brain injury
5. __________	Caregiver role strain	e. R/T breast engorgement
6. __________	Acute pain	f. R/T changes in appearance, lifestyle, role, and response of others secondary to severe trauma
7. __________	Imbalanced nutrition: Less than body requirements	g. R/T inadequate sensory stimulation
8. __________	Readiness for enhanced spiritual well-being	h. R/T dysphagia secondary to cerebral palsy
9. __________	Interrupted family processes	i. R/T right hip pain secondary to hip replacement
10. __________	Powerlessness	j. No etiology

Telephone Report

Nurses sometimes contact clinicians about a client by telephone—for example, when there is a medical emergency or when there is a significant or noteworthy change in the client's condition.

The nurse caring for Mr. Yang contacts the attending physician by telephone about a change in Mr. Yang's condition. Here is what the nurse reports to the physician, referred to as a *telephone report*:

> *Hello, Dr. Suki. This is Tamima, the RN caring for Mr. Yang, a 64-year-old man, in Room 1758. He was admitted for angina. He has a history of myocardial infarction, hypertension, atherosclerosis, and hypercholesterolemia. He is on nitroglycerin, chewable aspirin, and hydromorphone IV push PRN. His vital signs are unstable: his temp is 99.1, blood pressure is 177 over 120, shallow respirations of 24, and an irregular bounding pulse of 100. He coded* 10 minutes ago and I called the Rapid Response Team† since he is Full Code; they are currently responding to him. They suspect that he is having a myocardial infarction. Please come up to see him as soon as you can. Also, please let me know how you would like to proceed with this situation.*

*Coded (or coding) refers to a cardiopulmonary arrest that has happened (or is happening) to a client in a hospital or clinic, requiring a team of providers (Rapid Response Team) to rush to the specific location and begin immediate resuscitative efforts.

†Rapid Response Team = RRT

Documentation of Telephone Report

After completing the telephone report, the nurse documents the date, the time, the person called, the person who received the information, what information was given, and what information was received. Figure 3-2 shows the documentation of the telephone report about Mr. Yang.

Figure 3-3: Documentation of Telephone Report

09-25-13 1350 Dan Yang. Coded, RRT informed. T 99.1, BP 177/120, RR 24, irregular bounding pulse 100. MI suspected. Dr. Suki notified via phone. --T. Suleiman, RN

Telephone Order

In response to telephone reports, clinicians usually change medication and other orders for the client. Here is the attending physician's response to the nurse's report about Mr. Yang, referred to as a *telephone order* (T.O.). Note that spoken delivery of medication orders differs in some ways from written orders.

> *Hello, Tamima. From your brief summary on Mr. Yang in Room 1758, discontinue the hydromorphone IV and start infusing 5 milligrams per hour of morphine continuous IV. I believe RRT has him on high flow oxygen at this time and have intubated him. Administer 1 milligram of nitroglycerin sublingually immediately. Closely monitor his ECG* pattern. Monitor his vitals every 10 minutes. I am currently in the operating room, but will send the resident physician there in 5 minutes and come in 20 minutes once I am done with the critical part of this surgery.*

*ECG or electrocardiogram = the tracing made by an electrocardiograph (electrocardiograph = instrument for recording the electrical activity of the heart, used especially in diagnosing changes in heart rate and rhythm)

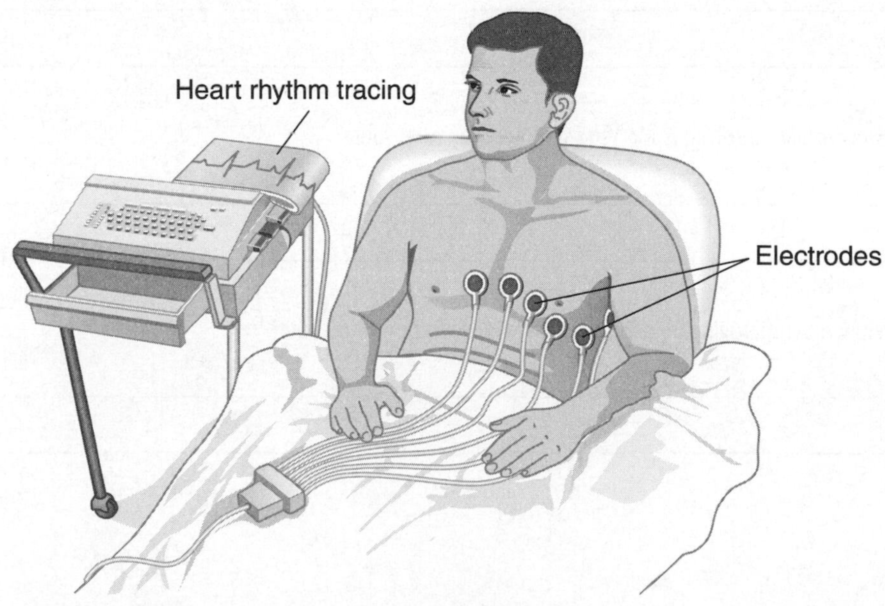

Figure 3-4: ECG

Documentation of Telephone Order

The nurse must document telephone orders from the physician. Figure 3-3 shows the nurse's documentation of the telephone order about Mr. Yang, referred to as a *telephone order report.*

Figure 3-5: Telephone Order Report

1. D/C hydromorphone IV
2. Start morphine 5 mg/hr continuous IV stat
3. Administer nitroglycerin 1 mg sublingually stat
4. Closely monitor ECG pattern
5. Monitor vitals q10 min

09-25-13 1410
T.O. from Dr. Suki /Tamima Suleiman, RN

▶ Activity 3.9: Understanding Telephone Order Report

Answer the following questions based on the telephone order report about Mr. Yang.

1. What medications are now ordered for Mr. Yang?

____

____

2. Which medication for Mr. Yang is discontinued?

____

____

3. How much morphine is Mr. Yang given and by what route?

____

____

4. How much nitroglicerin is Mr. Yang given now and by what route?

____

____

5. How often does the nurse check Mr. Yang's vitals now? How often did the nurse check the vitals in Scenario #3? How often does the nurse check the vitals in Documentation of Client Care: Progress Note later in the chapter? Why is there a difference in the frequency, do you think?

____

____

____

____

____

6. What else does the nurse monitor in the care of Mr. Yang?

____

____

Documentation of Client Care: Progress Note

At the end of the day shift, the nurse documents the care that was given to the client in the form of a progress note. Here is the progress note about the care that was provided to Mr. Yang.

Progress Note

Identify Problem(s)

Severe chest pain, decreased oxygen level, unstable vital signs, ineffective breathing*

Desired Outcome(s)

Pt will report chest pain at 3 or below on a scale of 0 to 10 within 1 hour of analgesic administration.

Pt will have O_2 sats at 92% and above throughout the shift.

Pt will have stable vital signs throughout the shift: blood pressure (120/80), pulse (60–100), respiration rate (12–20), temperature (98.6°), and O_2 sats (95–100%).

Pt will have respiration rate of 14–20 and will not use accessory muscles to breathe throughout the shift.†

Evaluation

VS before RRT unstable: BP 177/120, P 100, RR 24, T 99. Client coded and RRT was alerted. After RRT, VS were: BP 152/97, P 88, RR 17, T 98.8. Pt currently on morphine at 5 mg/hr. He is currently on 5L of medium flow oxygen and intubated.‡ Nitroglycerin 1mg was administered sublingually during period of unresponsiveness. Pt was weak and frightened after MI occurred. He spoke very little, and spoke softly and slowly. Pt is NPO. Pt on bed rest and his movement is currently restricted. He has a pressure-relieving mattress§ and is wearing a sequential compression device.*f* Breathing is still shallow but within normal range. Pt denies nausea and vomiting and his bowel sounds are hypoactive.¶ Pt states pain is a 2 on a scale of 0 to 10. ECG reveals dysrhythmias# present. Hmong language interpreter was called during attending physician's update. His wife and shaman are unhappy with intubation and requested that it be removed due to cultural beliefs that invasive procedures may cause the man's soul to leave his body. Attending physician explained need for intubation right now, but discussed possibility of discontinuing intubation if pt's respiratory status improves in 8 hours. Wife and shaman agreed to plan. As family believes illness is due to Mr. Yang's soul having left his body, shaman will perform a soul-calling ceremony in Mr. Yang's home.

Plan

Continue to monitor client health status and progress. Closely monitor his ECG pattern. Monitor his vitals every 20 minutes. Continue to administer medications per MAR. Provide quiet, healing environment for pt and maintain on bed rest to promote well-being. Limit visitors to immediate family members only at this time. Discuss plan of care with client and wife. Encourage pt to inform nurse of any concerns regarding his health and care.

*ineffective breathing = shallow, irregular in rhythm, and either slow or rapid in rate

†effective breathing = deep regular in rhythm, and within the normal range of 12–20 respirations per minute

‡intubated = tube is inserted into trachea to allow passage of air

§Use of a pressure-relieving mattress limits the development of pressure ulcers.

*f*Wearing a sequential compression device prevents the development of deep vein thrombosis (DVT), which is a blood clot in the deep veins of the leg or pelvis.

¶hypoactive = extremely soft and infrequent bowel sounds (e.g., 5 per minute); less than normally active

#dysrhythmia = abnormal rhythm in electrical impulses in the heart

▶ Activity 3.10: Providing Culturally Competent Care

Determine your answers to the following questions based on the care provided to Mr. Yang.

1. What concerns do Mr. Yang's wife and the shaman have about the intubation? How does the physician respond to their concern? Does the physician's response reflect culturally competent care? If so, in what ways?

____

____

____

____

____

2. Scenario #3 reported that a shaman was on his way to see Mr. Yang in the hospital and that a soul-calling ceremony was being planned. At the time of the progress note, the nurse reports that the ceremony will be performed in Mr. Yang's house. What do you think happened? Does the progress note reflect culturally competent care? If so, in what ways?

____

____

____

____

____

3. Does the plan (of care) in the progress note reflect culturally competent care of Mr. Yang? Why or why not?

____

____

____

____

____

Expansion of Documentation of Client Care: Characteristics of Effective Documentation

To document accurately and effectively, use medical/nursing abbreviations and acronyms and other concise words and expressions.

Medical/Nursing Abbreviations and Acronyms

Use only abbreviations, acronyms, and symbols that are accepted by the health care facility where you work. Leave off the period at the end of abbreviations. Note that some abbreviations have more than 1 meaning. For example, *d/c* could mean "discharge" or "discontinue." You have already seen some of these abbreviations.

▶ Activity 3.11: Understanding Abbreviations and Acronyms

Match the abbreviation or acronym with the corresponding word or phrase. Write the abbreviation or acronym in the correct blank. The first one has been done for you.

Abbreviations

½	L	hr/h
drsg	SOB	approx
BM	ROM	sm
amt	$\bar{s}$	$\bar{c}$
×3 days	c/o	fld
OOB	pericare	sol
Ⓡ	D&C	H_2O_2
Ⓛ	vag	

Word/Phrases

1. OOB out of bed
2. __________ right
3. __________ range of motion
4. __________ left
5. __________ complains of
6. __________ shortness of breath
7. __________ dressing
8. __________ for 3 days
9. __________ bowel movement
10. __________ without
11. __________ approximately
12. __________ hydrogen peroxide
13. __________ liters

14. __________ solution

15. __________ fluid

16. __________ dilation and curettage

17. __________ perineal care

18. __________ with

19. __________ one half

20. __________ small

21. __________ amount

22. __________ vagina

23. __________ hours

Concise Wording

Be concise in documenting nursing care. Concise writing is brief and to-the-point. It is often grammatically incomplete. Change full sentences into thought units. Eliminate words that are understood by the context. For example, do not include the client's name or the word *client* or *patient*. In addition, include only words that carry meaning. Eliminate words that have a grammatical function only, such as the verb "to be" (*is/are*), "helping" verbs (*is/are* with -ing verbs), and possessive adjectives (*his/her*).

The following are examples of full sentences:

Full Sentences: "The client is perspiring profusely. His respirations are shallow and occur at a rate of 28 per minute. Diffuse coarse crackles heard throughout lungs."

To change these sentences into thought units, all unnecessary words are eliminated:

Thought Units: "Perspiring profusely. Respirations shallow, crackles, 28/min."

Note that each thought unit ends with a period even though the thought unit is not a complete sentence.

Abbreviations and acronyms are also used to shorten the text. For example, instead of writing out complete phrases, such as "shortness of breath," use SOB, and for "complains of," use c/o:

Full Sentence: "The client complains of shortness of breath."

Thought Unit: "c/o SOB."

▶ Activity 3.12: Understanding Concise Wording

Match the more concise thought unit with the corresponding sentence. Write the letter of the thought unit in the correct blank. The first one has been done for you.

Complete Sentence	Thought Unit
1. ___h___ He is able to abduct right arm to shoulder height.	a. Full ROM Ⓡ wrist and fingers
2. ________ He is unable to flex right elbow.	b. Warm, moist palms
3. ________ He has full range of motion in right wrist and fingers.	c. No BM
4. ________ Mr. A tells you that he took a long time to void and that he had pain while voiding.	d. 10 min duration
5. ________ He stated that he flushed urine down the toilet.	e. Unable to flex Ⓡ elbow
6. ________ The pain lasted 10 minutes.	f. States that he voided with difficulty
7. ________ He has not moved his bowels.	g. Discarded urine by self
8. ________ The palms of her hands are warm and sweaty.	h. Able to abduct Ⓡ arm to shoulder height
9. ________ Baby V took 2 ounces of Similac.	i. 30 mL clear fluid removed
10. ________ The baby was sleeping.	j. Legs in alignment
11. ________ Her hips, knees, and ankles are not turned–either outward or inward.	k. Similac–60 mL taken
12. ________ Mr. F passes a lot of gas while he is expelling the enema.	l. Sm amt bleeding from vag
13. ________ Her respirations are below 16 breaths per minute.	m. Sleeping
14. ________ One ounce of clear fluid was removed through the needle.	n. Resp less than 16
15. ________ There is a small amount of blood coming from the vagina.	o. Expelling flatus

Communication Skills: Assessing Client's Pain

In order to obtain important health information from clients, such as a information about pain, nurses use various interviewing techniques. Read the dialog between the nurse and Mr. Yang, which takes place at the beginning of the day shift. Notice the various interviewing techniques that the nurse uses to gather data from the client about his pain.

Note: Expressions that are underlined in the dialog are included in Activity 3.2: Understanding Client Talk—Describing Symptoms and Feelings.

Dialog between Nurse and Mr. Yang

Nurse: *Good afternoon, Mr. Yang. How are you doing?*

Mr. Yang: *I'm fine. (breathing through clenched teeth)*

Nurse: *You say you're fine, but you seem to be in pain. Can you tell me more about how you are feeling right now?*

Mr. Yang: *I'm doing better than last night.*

Nurse: *I'm glad that you are feeling better, but are you in any pain right now? (nurse pulls a chair closer to the bed and takes a seat)*

Mr. Yang: *Yes, a little. (biting lower lip)*

Nurse: *Tell me more. Where is your pain?*

Mr. Yang: *In my chest.*

Nurse: *On a scale of 0 to 10, with 0 no pain and 10 the worst pain you can imagine, how would you rate your pain?*

Mr. Yang: *It's about a 5. It's not too bad. Earlier today the pain was killing me. But the medication helped . . .*

Nurse: *Tell me what your pain usually feels like.*

Mr. Yang: *It's a throbbing, burning feeling in my chest that causes tightness.*

Nurse: *Do you feel the chest pain radiating or moving to other parts of your body?*

Mr. Yang: *Sometimes I feel the pain in my shoulder, too.*

Nurse: *How long does the pain usually last?*

Mr. Yang: *Sometimes it lasts 10 minutes; other times up to 30 minutes. It just depends on how hard I'm working.*

Nurse: *What triggers or causes the pain? (leans in)*

Mr. Yang: *Well, when I work long hours at the restaurant and it gets too hot and busy in the kitchen, I get breathless and a little dizzy. I start breathing harder and then my chest begins to hurt. I have to sit down, but I can't. I have no time. I have to pay my bills. . . (rubbing palms together)*

Nurse: *As I understand it, the pressure at work makes the pain worse and makes it harder for you to get your work done. Is that correct?*

Mr. Yang: Yes.

Nurse: What relieves your pain or helps make it go away when you are at work?

Mr. Yang: Well, I take some aspirin, sit down, and let the fan blow on my face with a wet towel on my forehead. Sometimes I also rock back and forth to feel better. Lately my back has also been hurting . . . (trails off, but flexes back and makes facial grimace)

Nurse: I'm sorry, I didn't understand the last part of what you said, but you seem to be uncomfortable. Could you repeat that?

Mr. Yang: My back has been feeling stiff and tight.

Nurse: I see. Is there anything else that helps to relieve your pain?

Mr. Yang: Yes, I feel better when cupping is done on my chest to relieve the pressure and my fingers are pricked to release bad blood.

Nurse: From what I hear you say, the traditional treatments of cupping and pricking provide some relief to the pain. Is that correct?

Mr. Yang: Yes.

Nurse: I'm glad to hear that. I have just one more question for you. What do you fear most about your pain?

Mr. Yang: (Staring out the window, deep in thought) I fear that the pain will get so bad that I can no longer work. The restaurant supports my family, and times have been tough lately. I'm afraid that I will become dependent on painkillers. And what if I don't make it? . . . (watery eyes)

Nurse: I understand that your health situation has been quite challenging for you and your family.

Mr. Yang: (silence)

Nurse: So, I would like to wrap up our conversation now, but before we finish, let me make sure that I have noted everything that you have said about your pain: Right now your pain is about a 5 on a scale of 0 to 10. Your pain is usually a throbbing, burning feeling in your chest that causes tightness, and sometimes the pain moves to your shoulder. More recently your back has been hurting, too. The pain in your chest usually lasts 10 minutes, but can last as long as 30 minutes. Getting overexerted in the restaurant seems to trigger the pain, but when you sit down and cool off, it gets better. Traditional treatments also seem to help. You also seem concerned about how the pain will affect your ability to work in the restaurant. Is there anything else you would like to add?

Mr. Yang: Yes, I want to know what is wrong with me and what the doctors can do to help me get well.

Nurse: After the cardiac consult this afternoon, the physicians will hopefully come up with a solution that will provide long-lasting relief. In the meantime, during my shift, I will do my best to make sure that your pain is controlled and that you feel comfortable and well taken care of.

Mr. Yang: Thank you very much. (smiling)

▶ Activity 3.13: Analyzing Effectiveness of Communication

Determine your answers to the following questions about the effectiveness of the nurse's interview of Mr. Yang about his pain.

1. Is the nurse able to obtain information from Mr. Yang about his experiences of pain? Why or why not?

____

____

2. What are some examples of different types of questions the nurse asks Mr. Yang about his experiences of pain?

____

____

____

3. Does the nurse encounter any obstacles in obtaining information from Mr. Yang? If so, how does the nurse overcome the obstacle(s)?

____

____

____

4. Why does it take Mr. Yang a little while before he states that he is in pain?

____

____

5. Was the nurse effective in her response to the traditional remedies that Mr. Yang talked about? Why or why not?

____

____

____

Expansion of Dialog: Taking a Pain History

To manage pain effectively, the client's pain must first be accurately assessed. In addition to observing the client's physiologic and behavioral responses to pain, the nurse must take a pain history as part of the assessment process. Information about all aspects of the pain is gathered during the interview.

In the dialog between the nurse and Mr. Yang, the nurse takes a pain history. The nurse asks questions regarding the location and radiation of the pain; its intensity, quality, and duration; any precipitating and alleviating factors; and the meaning of the pain for the client.

▶ Activity 3.14: Identifying Questions about Pain

Review the dialog between the nurse and Mr. Yang. Write down the question (or statement) that the nurse uses to get information about each of the following aspects of pain. If the aspect is not represented in the dialog, write "none." Then, write down another question (or statement) that could be used to get information about the same aspect of pain. The first one has been done for you.

Aspect of Pain	Question from Dialog; Additional Question
Location	"Where is your pain?" "Can you tell me where you feel pain?"
Intensity	______
Radiating quality	______
Movement	______
Time of onset	______
Duration	______
Constancy	______
Precipitating factors	______
Alleviating factors	______
Associated symptoms	______
Effects on activities of daily living (ADLs)	______
Past pain experiences	______
Personal meaning of pain	______
Coping resources	______
Affective response	______

Expansion of Dialog: Rating and Describing Pain

Clients are often asked to rate their pain on a scale of intensity, with 0 representing "no pain" and 10 the "worst pain possible." For most clients, this is the easiest and most reliable way for them to measure their experience of pain. Shown is the complete set of word descriptors for different ratings of pain.

Pain Rating Scale

0	1	2	3	4	5	6	7	8	9	10
No pain		Mild pain			Moderate pain			Severe pain		Worst pain possible

▶ Activity 3.15: Understanding Client's Rating of Pain

Mr. Yang is asked to rate his pain several times during his stay at the hospital: when he is first admitted at night (see Scenario #3), at the beginning of the day shift (see Dialog between Nurse and Mr. Yang), and at the end of the day shift (see Documentation of Client Care: Progress Note).

Review Scenario #3, the dialog, and the Progress Note, in that order, and write down Mr. Yang's ratings of his pain, as well as the descriptors from the traditional pain rating scale. Then determine your answers to the questions that follow.

Ratings of Pain

<u>Scenario #3</u>

____

____

<u>Dialog</u>

____

____

<u>Progress Note</u>

____

____

Questions about Mr. Yang's Ratings of Pain

1. Why is there a difference between Mr. Yang's rating of his pain at the time of his admission to the hospital and at the time of the interview with the nurse, the following morning?

____

____

2. Why does Mr. Yang say he is fine during the interview but then rate his pain at a 5, indicating "moderate pain"?

____

____

3. Why is there a difference between Mr. Yang's rating of his pain from the time of the interview to the progress note, several hours later?

____

____

Describing Pain

It is clients, not nurses, who are best able to describe their experience of pain. Nurses must allow clients to express, in their own words, how they are experiencing pain, and nurses need to record the exact words that clients use to describe their pain.

▶ Activity 3.16: Understanding Client's Descriptions of Pain

In the dialog with the nurse, what words does Mr. Yang use to describe his pain? List them in the space provided. Look back at Scenario #3 and add any additional words that Mr. Yang used to describe his pain when he was first admitted to the hospital.

Descriptive Words

____

____

____

____

____

Use a nursing textbook, an English language medical dictionary, or online resources to locate 8–10 other adjectives that are used to describe the **sensory** (or physiological) experience of pain and 8–10 words that are used to describe the **affective** (or emotional) experience of pain. Categorize the words based on the intensity of the pain they represent (**mild, moderate, severe,** or **worst pain possible**). Then, identify those words that describe pattern of pain, including onset, duration, and constancy of pain. Mark those words with (**P**) for pattern.

Sensory Words

Mild	Moderate	Severe	Worst Pain Possible

Affective Words

Mild	Moderate	Severe	Worst Pain Possible

Expansion of Dialog: Interviewing Skills (Open-Ended Questions, Focused Questions, Probes, Paraphrases, Requests for Clarification, Discrepancy Tests, Summaries, and Closing)

Interviewing skills are used by nurses to gather information from a client about past and present illnesses, the client's understanding of the current illness, the client's work and family situation, and other psychosocial information about the client that could be relevant. This information is used to assess the client's situation and ongoing needs and to determine appropriate nursing goals.

Open-Ended Questions

Open-ended questions give clients options regarding how to respond and what to say. They require more than a yes/no answer or minimal response. They encourage clients to describe a problem or issue in their own words. In contrast, **closed questions** require a 1- or 2-word response. **Yes/no questions** are 1a type of closed questions.

Examples: "How are you today?"

"How have you been?"

"How is everything going?"

"What brings you in today?"

"What seems to be the problem?"

In addition, some open-ended questions are stated as commands:

Example: "Tell me about (your problem, family, work, etc.)."

Open-ended questions are especially useful at the beginning of an interview or at the beginning of a new topic. They are preferable to closed questions because they encourage clients to talk, sometimes revealing important information that might otherwise be missed. In some situations, however, they may not be appropriate, such as in an emergency room when focused information is needed quickly.

▶ Activity 3.17: Identifying Open-Ended Questions

Identify each of the following questions as either open-ended or closed. (For the closed questions, consider when they would be appropriate to use.) The first one has been done for you.

1. "How are you feeling?"	1. Open
2. "Are you feeling pain?"	2. ______________________
3. "Tell me about the pain."	3. ______________________
4. "What are you doing for the pain?"	4. ______________________
5. "Are you taking any medication?"	5. ______________________
6. "Are you available at 11 o'clock for your next appointment?"	6. ______________________
7. "When are you available for your next appointment?"	7. ______________________
8. "Are you exercising regularly?"	8. ______________________
9. "How often do you exercise?"	9. ______________________
10. "Tell me about your physical activity."	10. ______________________

▶ Activity 3.18: Analyzing Dialog for Open-Ended Questions

Look back at the dialog between the nurse and Mr. Yang. Identify any examples of open-ended questions in the dialog. What is the effect of the open-ended question(s)? Are there other instances where the nurse could have used open-ended questions?

____

____

____

____

____

▶ Activity 3.19: Asking Open-Ended Questions

Practice asking open-ended questions of the client. Revise the closed questions on the left, so they are open-ended. The first one has been done for you.

Nurse's Closed Question	Nurse's Open-Ended Alternative
1. "Where is the pain?"	1. "Tell me about the pain."
2. "Did you have a good week?"	2. ____________________
3. "Do you have children?"	3. ____________________
4. "You look sad. Are you depressed?"	4. ____________________
5. "Have you eaten today?"	5. ____________________

Focused Questions

Focused questions move beyond introductory, open-ended questions and narrow the range of inquiry to a particular topic. They frequently ask for more information or history about a specific issue or problem. In that way, they limit the range of options the client has for responding, but they still encourage more than a 1-word response. As a result, focused questions share characteristics of both closed and open-ended questions.

Examples: "You only mentioned your family briefly. Can you tell me more about them?"

"You complained about anxiety the last time I saw you. How is your anxiety now?"

"How has your foot been this week? Last week it was giving you a lot of trouble."

"Tell me about the pain in your arm."

The difference between open-ended questions and focused questions can be subtle. For example, in the open-ended question, "Tell me about the pain," the location of the pain is not identified, but in the focused question, "Tell me about the pain *in your arm*," it is. Open-ended questions do not assume any prior knowledge of a problem. Focused questions, on the other hand, ask about specific problems or issues that have already been identified.

▶ Activity 3.20: Analyzing Dialog for Focused Questions

Look back at the dialog between the nurse and Mr. Yang. Identify any examples of focused questions in the dialog. What is the effect of the focused question(s)? Are there other instances where the nurse could have used focused questions?

____

____

____

____

____

▶ Activity 3.21: Asking Focused Questions

Practice asking focused questions of the client. For each open-ended question on the left, write a follow-up question that is focused. The first one has been done for you.

Nurse's Open-Ended Question	Nurse's Focused Question
1. "Tell me about the pain."	1. "Tell me about the pain in your leg."
2. "How have you been this week?"	2. ____________________
3. "Tell me about your family."	3. ____________________
4. "You look sad. How are you feeling?"	4. ____________________
5. "What have you been eating lately?"	5. ____________________

Probes

Probes go beyond focused questions; they ask for further detail about a specific topic. They can be open-ended, focused, or closed-ended questions. They do not have to be stated as questions; they can be words or phrases, as long as they are used to gain additional information about the same topic. Some probes are general; others are specific.

Examples of Probes:

General Probes

"Tell me more."

"And . . ."

"Um-hmm" (followed by silence)

"How do you feel about that?"

"Is there anything you left out?"

Specific Probes "How long have you had the pain in your leg?"

"Have you been skipping meals lately?"

"Have you needed any medication to get to sleep at night?"

"What are you doing for your cough?"

▶ Activity 3.22: Analyzing Dialog for Probes

Look back at the dialog between the nurse and Mr. Yang. Identify any examples of probes, both general and specific, in the dialog. What is the effect of the probes? Are there other instances where the nurse could have used probes?

____

____

____

____

____

Paraphrases

Paraphrasing means putting into your own words what someone else has said. Paraphrasing lets the client know you are listening. Paraphrasing is important in an interview because it confirms to the client that the nurse has been listening, helping to build trust and rapport between the client and nurse. It also gives the nurse the opportunity to verify his or her understanding of what the client has said and the client the opportunity to add or clarify anything that might have been misunderstood.

Example:

Client's Statement	**Nurse's Paraphrase**
"I've had the arthritis for a long time, but it doesn't seem to get any worse."	"So, although you've had it quite a while, it's about the same?"

When paraphrasing, the nurse has to be careful not to change the client's meaning even though different words are used. Paraphrases are ineffective if they change the client's meaning. Compare the following examples of effective and ineffective paraphrasing:

Examples:

Client's Statement	**Effective Paraphrase**
"It doesn't seem to get any worse."	"It's about the same."
	Ineffective Paraphrases
	"It's probably better."
	"It's hard to tell if it changes."

In some ways, paraphrasing is similar to reflection because the focus is on giving back to the client what the client has said, but there are also several differences. With reflection, the nurse gives back to the client *feelings* that the client has stated or implied, whereas with paraphrasing, the nurse gives back *information* that the client has stated. Also, in reflection, the nurse often uses the client's exact words and phrases, whereas in paraphrasing, the nurse changes the client's words. Finally, the purpose of reflection is to encourage the client to further explore feelings, but with paraphrasing, the purpose is to check the nurse's understanding of information.

As in reflecting, many paraphrases begin with "you." The use of "you" statements is appropriate because the nurse's intent is to clarify information that the client has stated, in contrast to "I" statements (see the section on "I" statements in Chapter One), where the focus is on the nurse owning his or her own feelings and concerns.

If the nurse is unsure about the client's meaning, the paraphrase could begin, *"I think that you . . . "* or *"Sounds like . . . ,"* as shown here.

Example: "Sounds like it's about the same."

Too much paraphrasing, however, can interrupt the flow of conversation and suggest to the client that he or she is not being listened to. Rather than paraphrase everything the client says, the nurse can also wait until the interview is over and then summarize the main points of what the client has said. At that point the nurse can confirm what she or he has understood and the client can add any missing information.

▶ Activity 3.23: Analyzing Dialog for Paraphrasing

Look back at the dialog between the nurse and Mr. Yang. Identify any examples of paraphrasing in the dialog. What is the effect of the paraphrasing? Are there other instances where the nurse could have used paraphrasing?

___

___

___

___

___

▶ Activity 3.24: Paraphrasing

Practice paraphrasing what the client has said. For each statement on the left, read the unacceptable paraphrase by the nurse. Write down why the paraphrase is unacceptable. Then, write an acceptable alternative. The first one has been done for you.

Client's Statement	Nurse's Paraphrase
1. "I haven't been sleeping well. I can't sleep at night and then I can't get up in the morning."	1a. Unacceptable: "Sounds like you're depressed." Reason why unacceptable: does not rephrase what client has said 1b. Acceptable: "You've been having trouble sleeping."
2. "The doctor told me to take 1 pill twice a day until the pills ran out, but I felt better the next day, so I stopped."	2a. Unacceptable: "You did not understand the doctor." Reason why unacceptable: ____________ 2b. Acceptable: ____________ ____________ ____________
3. "I don't believe that smoking is bad for you. I've smoked a pack a day for 20 years."	3a. Unacceptable: "Maybe you'll believe that smoking is dangerous when you have a heart attack!" Reason why unacceptable: ____________ 3b. Acceptable: ____________ ____________ ____________
4. "My child has a fever and sore throat. What should I do?"	4a. Unacceptable: "That sounds like a cold. Don't worry about it." Reason why unacceptable: ____________ 4b. Acceptable: ____________ ____________ ____________
5. "I'd like to lose some weight, but the holidays are coming up."	5a. Unacceptable: "You should watch what you eat if you really want to lose weight." Reason why unacceptable: ____________ 5b. Acceptable: ____________ ____________ ____________

Requests for Clarification

Sometimes in an interview the client will say or do something that is confusing or unclear to the nurse. When that happens, the nurse can either ask the client immediately for clarification or wait until later in the interview or for another time to ask, depending on the situation and the state of the client.

Examples: "I'm not sure I understood that completely. Could you repeat it?"

"I missed the last few words you said."

"I don't follow you. Can you say it another way?"

▶ Activity 3.25: Analyzing Dialog for Clarification Requests

Look back at the dialog between the nurse and Mr. Yang. Identify any examples of clarification requests in the dialog. What is the effect of the clarification request? Are there other instances where the nurse could have asked for clarification?

____

____

____

____

____

Discrepancy Tests

Sometimes clients are inconsistent in the information they give you; other times there is a discrepancy between the information they give you and the feelings they convey through their body language. For example, a client might tell you her family visits every day, but later the client complains of feeling lonely. Another client who is writhing in pain might tell you he feels fine. Neither of these messages makes sense because the verbal and nonverbal messages are inconsistent with each other.

If the nurse decides to explore the discrepancy, the nurse should first summarize the discrepancy and then ask the client to clarify or explain what the client is thinking or feeling. By summarizing what the nurse has observed, the nurse remains nonjudgmental, thereby encouraging the client to explore his or her feelings more openly. By asking for clarification, the nurse gives the client the opportunity to become more aware of his or her feelings, and in the process the nurse can learn from the client's understanding and explanation of the discrepancy.

▶ Activity 3.26: Analyzing Dialog for Discrepancy Tests

Look back at the dialog between the nurse and Mr. Yang. Identify any examples of testing discrepancies in the dialog. What is the effect of testing discrepancies? Are there other instances where the nurse could have tested a discrepancy?

____

____

____

____

____

▶ Activity 3.27: Testing Discrepancies

Practice testing the client's discrepancies. For each of the discrepancies on the left, write down how the nurse could explore the discrepancy with the client. The first one has been done for you.

Client's Discrepancy	Nurse's Response
1. A client is sitting in a clinic, waiting to be seen. The client seems preoccupied: He is wringing his hands and his eyes are watery. When asked how he feels, he says, "Just fine."	1. "You say you're just fine, but you seem preoccupied. How do you really feel?"
2. A client is grossly overweight. When asked about his diet, he claims that he does not eat much and always eats healthy food.	2. ______________________
3. A client in the hospital says that her family visits regularly. Later, the client says she always feels lonely.	3. ______________________
4. A client says that he does not smoke, yet his clothes smell of smoke and his teeth are heavily stained with nicotine.	4. ______________________
5. You ask an elderly client what her address is, and the client responds, "1327 Marshall." Later, the client writes down "2713 Marshall."	5. ______________________

Summaries

At the end of the interview or at a logical breaking point during the interview, it is helpful to summarize what the client has said so far. Like paraphrasing, summarizing involves putting what the client has said into your own words. However, in paraphrasing, the nurse usually puts one point into his or her own words, whereas in summarizing, the nurse condenses an entire conversation. Also, in summarizing, not everything the client has said is included. Include only the essence of what the client has said, such as relevant facts and feelings, as well as the essence of what the client has not said, such as implied feelings. In addition, any discrepancies between what the client has said and done and any untouched areas of discussion should be included. Finally, the summary should end with giving the client the opportunity to add information.

As in paraphrasing, summarizing confirms to the client that the nurse has been listening and wants to understand, but it also gives the client the opportunity to clarify anything the nurse may not have understood. Also, clients sometimes wait until the last minute to give the nurse the most important information, so by summarizing what has been said so far and giving clients the opportunity to add anything they wish, summarizing can help bring out important additional information. Finally, summarizing gives the nurse the opportunity to pull together pieces of information for future recording or charting.

This is a description of an interview with a client:

Interview: A nurse has been talking with a 37-year-old male who will be discharged this afternoon following a brain aneurysm rupture. Their discussion covered the need for a follow-up visit to the clinic; a review of his recovery plan, including activity, exercise, diet, and rest; and his perceptions of the family's response to his illness. He also voiced concerns about his sexual functioning to the nurse but not to his wife, and he has openly wondered about what effect his illness will have on his work as a mechanical engineer at an automanufacturing company.

Here is one way for the nurse to summarize the interview with this client:

Summary: "Let me see if I have everything we talked about. We reviewed your recovery plan and your family's response to your illness. You still have some concerns about its effects on your work as a mechanical engineer and your sexual relationship with your wife. However, you have not talked about it with her. Is there anything else?"

Note that in the summary, the nurse begins with the introductory phrase: "Let me see if I have everything we talked about." Introductory phrases help the client realize that the nurse is beginning a summary. Other introductory phrases are "As I understand it" and "From what you've said."

The nurse ends with a request for confirmation: "Is there anything else?" Requests for confirmation communicate the nurse's openness to any clarification or addition from the client. Another request for confirmation is "Is that it?"

Note that a summary is always shorter than the original interview. By contrast, a paraphrase is not necessarily shorter; indeed, it could be longer.

▶ Activity 3.28: Analyzing Dialog for Summarizing

1. Look back at the dialog between the nurse and Mr. Yang. Does the nurse summarize the interview? What is the effect of summarizing the interview?

2. Consider the summary without the introductory phrase and the request for confirmation. Would the summary be less effective as a result? Why or why not?

▶ Activity 3.29: Summarizing

For each of the case notes listed, write a summary of the interview in 1 or 2 sentences. The first one has been done for you.

Case Notes	Summary
1. A pregnant client came to the clinic at 24 weeks for a prenatal visit. She is experiencing fatigue, edema, and abdominal pain. She expresses concern about her baby's health and her performance at work.	1. "From what you have said, you're concerned about your baby's health and your own performance at work. You've been having some issues with edema, abdominal pain and fatigue. Is that correct?"
2. A teenage female client came to the school nurse and was anxious because she almost fainted in class. She has been experiencing a burning sensation while urinating and often sweats uncontrollably. She has never felt this way before and her friends suggested that she go home for the day. She is worried about missing her final exam.	2. ______________________________
3. A male client diagnosed with a tibia fracture cannot feel his feet and fingers. He complains of drowsiness, thirst, and a severe headache. His wife and 2 children have not been in to see him and he is concerned about their well-being.	3. ______________________________

Closing

At the end of an interview it is important to bring closure to the interaction. Closing an interview should be done smoothly so that the client does not feel rushed or cut off. A sudden, unannounced departure could create mistrust or provoke a sense of loss, especially if a personal bond was created during the interview. Some ways to acknowledge the end of an interview are as follows.

Examples: "Well, I see our time is nearly up. It's been nice talking with you."

"I have to finish in a minute."

"We need to wrap up now. I'll stop by tomorrow to see how you're doing."

"That's about all the time I have today—would you like another appointment?"

The last 2 examples offer the possibility of a continuation of the nurse–client relationship, initiated either by the nurse, as in, "I'll stop by tomorrow to see how you're doing," or by the client, who requests another appointment.

Sometimes it is best to announce at the beginning of an interview how long the interview will last. This strategy is especially helpful for student nurses, who may find that clients are reluctant to share information and feelings during the interview because of the short amount of time nursing students spend with clients.

▶ Activity 3.30: Opening and Closing an Interview

Determine your answers to the following questions.

1. Look back at the dialog between the nurse and Mr. Yang. Does the nurse close the interview? What is the effect of closing an interview?

____

____

____

____

2. As a student nurse, how could you begin an interview to let the client know how long it will last? Write out 1 or 2 possibilities.

____

____

____

____

3. As a student nurse, how would you close the interview to be consistent with your opening? Write out 1 or 2 possibilities.

____

____

____

____

4. When is it appropriate for a student nurse to offer the possibility of continuing the nurse–client relationship after the interview? What is the effect of offering such a possibility to a client?

____

____

____

____

Culture in Nursing: Culture and Pain Management

Cultural groups vary in their response to pain. Some clients may choose not to talk about their pain or to downplay it, like Mr. Yang, or they may describe their pain in ways the nurse does not understand. As a result, nurses can misunderstand a client's experience of pain and not provide adequate pain medication.

A client's rating of his or her pain is not always an adequate measure of pain. Some clients may rate their pain at 3 or 4, but state they cannot walk, dress, or participate in other activities of daily living. Or their behavioral response to pain—frowning and moaning—and changes in their vital signs may indicate much greater pain than their rating. As a result, nurses should not rely on just one way of assessing pain.

▶ Activity 3.31: Considering Culture and Pain Management

Determine your answers to the following questions.

1. How do people in your culture generally respond to pain? Why? What are the prevailing beliefs and attitudes toward pain in your culture?

____

____

2. What words or images do people generally use to describe pain in your culture?

____

____

3. Are there any concerns about the use of opioids for pain medication in your culture? If so, what are they? Why do people have these concerns?

____

____

4. Are there differences in the beliefs, attitudes, and behaviors in response to pain among different groups in your culture? If so, what are they?

____

____

5. As a future health care provider, do you have any concerns about assessing and managing your clients' pain? If so, explain.

____

____

Chapter Three Answer Key

Activity 3.1: Considering Traditional Beliefs and Practices

1. Answers will vary, but some of the categories of discussion could include work, lifestyle, health, beliefs and practices regarding health and health care, and language. Despite the information that Mr. Yang is Hmong, it is essential not to make assumptions about a client's beliefs and practices regarding health and health care based solely on a client's ethnicity or country of origin. Cultures change over time, especially as the larger context changes, and there is also considerable variation within any cultural group, based on a variety of factors. It is important not to stereotype or rely on generalizations about any cultural group in providing culturally competent care. When in doubt, ask a client about his or her cultural beliefs and practices. What is important is being aware of cultural differences and respectful and responsive to those differences.

   That said, with regard to Mr. Yang, there are some indicators of cultural beliefs and practices, as well as cultural change, in Scenario #3. Although there is no information about when Mr. Yang moved to the United States, Hmong fighters associated with the U.S. "Secret War" in Laos came to this country in the late 1970s; families began arriving in the early 1980s. As a man in his 60s, Mr. Yang most likely was involved in the war in Laos and came to the United States in his early 30s. It is also likely that because Mr. Yang grew up in Laos and left the country as an adult, he has had to make some major lifestyle changes to adjust to life in the United States, and he may hold onto some traditional beliefs and practices with respect to health and health care. He runs a restaurant that he co-owns with his brother, indicating some degree of adaptation and success in this country. Although Mr. Yang's health issues may be genetic, they may also be related to a change in lifestyle when he first moved to the United States due to easy access to unhealthy (fast) food and a more sedentary lifestyle, as indicated by hypercholesterolemia or the presence of excess cholesterol in the blood. Regarding traditional health care practices, Mr. Yang received the traditional treatments of cupping and pricking before he came to the hospital for chest pain. In addition, a shaman is on his way to see Mr. Yang, and a soul-calling ceremony is being planned. Finally, although Mr. Yang seems to speak and understand English without any difficulty, his wife speaks little English, so a Hmong interpreter is needed for consultations and updates.

2. In order to provide culturally competent care, the hospital and health care staff need to be respectful of traditional beliefs and practices of clients. However, because the priority is client safety, health care staff cannot allow any practices to take place in the hospital setting that could jeopardize the safety of the client. Thus, the soul-calling ceremony will not take place in the hospital but rather in the client's home.

3. Without professionally trained medical interpreters, clinicians will have difficulty getting an accurate medical history from clients. If clinicians are not able to determine what the problem is, they may not be able to provide proper treatment in a timely fashion. They may order unnecessary tests and the client may end up staying in the hospital longer than necessary. In addition, the client may be at a greater risk for medical errors. Although hospitals that receive federal funds have been required to provide interpreters under the Civil Rights Act since 2000, one study found that less than a fourth of U.S. hospitals have interpreters, and most of these interpreters have not received professional training. (Source: "Hospital interpreters bridge language gaps, lower risks." *USA Today*. Available online. URL: http://usatoday30.usatoday.com/news/health/2004-11-21-hospital-translators_x.htm. Posted on November 21, 2004.) A more recent study found that even when professionally trained interpreters are available, they are underused, which adversely affects the quality of health care that clients with limited English proficiency receive. (Source: Diamond, L. C., Y. Schenker, L. Curry, E. H. Bradley, and A. Fernandez. "Getting by: Underuse of interpreters by resident physicians." *Journal of General Internal Medicine* 24(February 2009):2, 256–262.) Physicians tend to rely on family members, including children, hospital staff who are not trained interpreters, their own limited proficiency in the client's native language, and gestures. (Source: "Study explores underuse of interpreters in hospitals." University

of California–San Francisco. Available online. URL: http://www.ucsf.edu/news/2009/01/4194/study-explores-underuse-interpreters-hospitals. Posted on January 30, 2009.)

It is not appropriate to rely on family members (especially children) or friends as interpreters. In addition to not having the proper training to serve as medical interpreters, family members may not always translate unwelcome information to the client, and clients may not want to reveal certain private information to their family members, especially children.

▶ Activity 3.2: Understanding Client Talk—Describing Symptoms and Feelings

1. The client was experiencing severe pain.
2. The client is concerned that he will develop an addiction to pain medication.
3. The client is concerned that he will die.
4. The client got very sick.
5. The client does not feel hungry.
6. The client's stomach has been causing her a lot of discomfort.
7. The client is vomiting everything he eats.
8. The client is coughing up blood.

11. __d__ black out	a. become sick with an illness
12. __e__ break out	b. restore to consciousness
13. __b__ bring to	c. recover from a serious illness
14. __a__ come down with	d. lose consciousness, faint
15. __c__ pull through	e. show a rash or other skin disorder

Medical/Nursing Vocabulary

acute (pain): pain that is sharp and intense and lasts less than 6 months

analgesics: drugs that reduce pain without causing loss of consciousness

angina: sudden brief attacks of chest pain that are the clinical manifestations of insufficient oxygen in the heart muscles

atherosclerosis: condition in which deposits of fats and minerals form on the walls of an artery and prevent blood from flowing easily

bed rest: confinement of a sick person to bed

cardiac catheterization: insertion of a tubular medical device (catheter) into the heart, to take samples of tissue or to check blood pressure

cardiac/telemetry: unit in the hospital for clients requiring treatment for heart disease or the detection and measurement of heart disease

cardiology consult: consultation with a doctor specializing in the heart, its action, and its diseases

chewable: able to be crushed with the teeth, as in chewable aspirin

complain (of): to speak about one's illness or symptoms

diaphoresis: perspiration that is excessive

dietician consult: consultation with a specialist in the study of diet, especially applying the principles of nutrition to diet

electrolytes: minerals such as sodium, calcium, potassium, chlorine, phosphate, and magnesium, that have an electric charge. They are found in the blood, urine, and body fluids. Maintaining the right balance of electrolytes helps the body's blood chemistry, muscle action, and other processes.

exertion: physical activity

health history: account of client's family and personal background with regard to past and present health

hypercholesterolemia: presence of excess cholesterol in the blood

intense: very strong

jugular venous distention: condition of having jugular veins that are abnormally enlarged or stretched out (as from internal pressure)

myocardial: pertaining to the middle layer of the heart, or cardiac muscle

myocardial infarction: acute episode of heart disease marked by the death or damage of heart muscle due to insufficient blood supply, characterized by chest pain; also referred to as a *heart attack*

over-the-counter: a class of medications that are available without a prescription

pain management: the process of alleviating or reducing pain to a level that the client can accept

platelet: a component of mammalian blood that contributes to blood clotting to stop bleeding

radiating (to): describes pain that is felt at its source but also spreads to nearby tissues

stress test: electrocardiographic test of heart function before, during, and after a controlled period of increasingly strenuous exercise (as on a treadmill)

tachycardia: heart rate that is too fast

triage: sorting of and allocation of treatment to clients (as in an emergency room) according to the urgency of their need for care

troponin: muscle proteins that, when combined with calcium ions, permit muscular contraction. The troponin test measures the levels of troponin T and troponin I in the blood, proteins that are released when the heart muscle has been damaged, as in a heart attack. The more damage there is to the heart, the greater the amount of troponin T and I there will be in the blood.

▶ Activity 3.3: Identifying Responses to Pain

Mr. Yang's Physiologic Responses

Scenario #3

diaphoresis (sweating)

weakness

increased pulse rate (tachycardia)

Dialog

breathless (dyspnea)

dizzy

breathes harder (labored breathing, hyperventilation)

Mr. Yang's Behavioral Responses

Scenario #3

None

Dialog

clenches teeth

bites lower lip

rubs the palms of his hands together

flexes back

makes facial grimace

rocks back and forth (to relieve pain)

watery eyes

Additional Physiologic Responses

increased blood pressure

increased respiration rate

pupil dilation

pallor

Additional Behavioral Responses

There are 3 main types of behavioral responses to pain:

1. vocalizations, such as moaning, groaning, crying, and screaming
2. facial expressions, such as eyes tightly shut or eyes open and somber
3. body movement, such as tossing and turning in bed and flinging the arms about

▶ Activity 3.4: Frequency of Administration

1. stat at once
2. PRN as needed
3. am morning
4. pm afternoon
5. # number
6. × times

7. ____BID____ twice a day
8. ____TID____ 3 times a day
9. ____QID____ 4 times a day
10. ____hr____ hour
11. ____qh____ every hour
12. ____q2h____ every 2 hours
13. ____q4h____ every 4 hours
14. ____q6h____ every 6 hours
15. ____HS____ at bedtime
16. ____qhs____ every night at bedtime
17. ____AC____ before meals
18. ____PC____ after meals
19. ____$\bar{c}$____ with
20. ____$\bar{s}$____ without

▶ Activity 3.5: Identifying Medication Orders, Labs, Tests, and Nursing Actions in Scenario #3

Medications

Nitroglycerin: decreases myocardial oxygen demand; 1 tablet stat

Chewable aspirin: decreases platelet activity and clot formation; 325 mg once

Hydromorphone: relieves pain; 1.5 mg IV push PRN q3–4hr

Oxygen: increases oxygenation; 2 liters via nasal cannula if O_2 sats fall below 90%

The additional information that is provided is as follows: amount of medication, route of medication, and frequency of administration, in that order.

Labs/Tests

CBC lab

electrolyte labs (also referred to as chemistry panel)

focused cardiac assessment

focused respiratory assessment

stress test

troponin labs

Nursing Actions*

take VS every 15 minutes until decrease in chest pain

maintain NPO status

perform focused cardiac assessment

perform focused respiratory assessment

*Note that consults are not included here, as they are not performed by a nurse or NAP.

▶ Activity 3.6: Plan of Care: Planning for Client's Care

1. Angina
2. MI (myocardial infarction), HTN (hypertension), atherosclerosis, and hypercholesterolemia
3. 1.5 mg every 3 or 4 hours
4. Every 15 minutes until decrease in chest pain
5. Focused cardiac, focused respiratory, VS q15 min

Nursing Diagnosis: Planning Culturally Competent Care for Mr. Yang

The intervention "Nurse will encourage client to express any concerns and ask questions about treatment and procedures, and will welcome participation of family members in such discussions by the end of shift" responds to Mr. Yang's cultural values and beliefs regarding health care. In many cultures, the family is involved in key decisions in the health care of a family member. By recognizing and respecting this characteristic of Hmong culture, this nursing intervention is responsive to Mr. Yang's cultural values and beliefs regarding health care and thus reflects culturally competent care.

▶ Activity 3.7: Nursing Diagnosis: Nursing Interventions and Desired Outcomes

Nursing Intervention	Desired Outcome
1. ____b____ Nurse will administer oxygen, as ordered by physician, throughout shift.	a. Client will report decreased anxiety by the end of shift.
2. ____c____ Nurse will assess pain, both using the pain rating scale and assessing for signs and symptoms, and administer pain medication as needed throughout shift.	b. Client will maintain oxygen saturation level greater than 90% throughout shift.
3. ____d____ Nurse will assess vital signs every 15 minutes throughout shift until there is a decrease in chest pain.	c. Client will report pain level of 3 (scale 0–10) within 1 hour of analgesic administration.
4. ____a____ Nurse will encourage client to express any concerns and ask questions about treatment and procedures, and will welcome participation of family members in such discussions by the end of shift.	d. Client will maintain stable vital signs throughout shift: blood pressure (120/80), pulse (60–100), respiration rate (12–20), temperature (98.6°), and O_2 sats (95–100%).

▸ Activity 3.8: Understanding Problems and Etiologies

Problem	Etiology
1. ___e___ Ineffective breastfeeding	a. R/T disruption of family routine secondary to hospitalization
2. ___i___ Impaired physical mobility	b. R/T unrelenting care requirements and physical disabilities secondary to stroke
3. ___g___ Impaired verbal communication	c. R/T to knowledge deficit: nonpharmacological pain management
4. ___f___ Disturbed body image	d. R/T increased dependency secondary to trauma brain injury
5. ___b___ Caregiver role strain	e. R/T breast engorgement
6. ___c___ Acute pain	f. R/T changes in appearance, lifestyle, role, and response of others secondary to severe trauma
7. ___h___ Imbalanced nutrition: Less than body requirements	g. R/T inadequate sensory stimulation
8. ___j___ Readiness for enhanced spiritual well-being	h. R/T dysphagia secondary to cerebral palsy
9. ___a___ Interrupted family processes	i. R/T right hip pain secondary to hip replacement
10. ___d___ Powerlessness	j. no etiology

▸ Activity 3.9: Understanding Telephone Order Report

1. morphine, nitroglycerin

2. hydromorphone

3. 5 mg (of morphine) per hour, on continuous IV

4. 1 mg (of nitroglycerin), under the tongue (sublingually)

5. Mr. Yang's vitals are checked every 10 minutes now. In Scenario #3, upon admission to the hospital, they were checked every 15 minutes, and in the progress note, toward the end of the shift, they are checked every 20 minutes. Mr. Yang was admitted to the hospital complaining of intense chest pain, and he also was experiencing tachycardia and jugular venous distension, so his vitals were checked every 15 minutes. At the time of the telephone order, Mr. Yang is having a myocardial infarction, so the vital signs are checked more frequently (every 10 minutes). At the time of the progress note, the client is more stable, so the vital signs are being checked slightly less often (every 20 minutes).

6. ECG pattern

▶ Activity 3.10: Providing Culturally Competent Care

1. Mr. Yang's wife and the shaman are unhappy with the intubation and have requested that it be removed due to cultural beliefs that invasive procedures may cause the man's soul to leave his body. The attending physician explained the need for intubation right now, but discussed the possibility of discontinuing intubation if Mr. Yang's respiratory status improved in 8 hours. The wife and shaman agreed to the plan. The physician's response indicates that the physician has listened to and acknowledged the family's concerns. However, at the same time, because the priority is client safety, the physician cannot immediately comply with the family's desire to have the tube removed. After 8 hours, the physician will reassess the client's respiratory status and, if it has sufficiently improved, may remove the intubation at that time. By listening to the family's concern about intubation and working out a compromise that the family accepts, the physician's response reflects culturally competent care.

2. Presumably, a compromise was reached between the health care staff and the family to minimize any excitement or exertion that the soul-calling ceremony might have caused for Mr. Yang that could have had adverse consequences. By including information about the soul-calling ceremony in the progress note, along with the family's belief that Mr. Yang's illness is due to his soul having left his body, the nurse acknowledges and respects the client's traditional health care beliefs and practices that may have cultural or spiritual implications for the client. Also, a Hmong language interpreter was called during the attending physician's update, indicating the importance given to the wife being informed about her husband's condition, as well as being included in discussions about treatment and procedures. In these ways, the progress note reflects culturally competent care.

3. The plan of care does not acknowledge traditional clan structure in Hmong culture, as visitors have been limited to immediate family members only. Although the goal is to promote a quiet, healing environment for the client, the restriction on visitors does not allow for extended family and clan members to visit Mr. Yang. In addition, only the wife has been included in a discussion about the client's plan of care, not extended family or clan members. (Note that because the grandchildren are under the age of 18, they are not included in the discussion.) Thus, although the plan of care acknowledges the importance of family in the care of Mr. Yang, family is restricted to immediate family members only, thus denying the participation of family as defined in traditional Hmong culture. For this reason, the plan does not reflect culturally competent care.

▶ Activity 3.11: Understanding Abbreviations and Acronyms

	Abbreviations	Words/Phrases
1.	OOB	out of bed
2.	Ⓡ	right
3.	ROM	range of motion
4.	Ⓛ	left
5.	c/o	complains of
6.	SOB	shortness of breath
7.	drsg	dressing
8.	× 3 days	for 3 days

9. BM bowel movement
10. $\overline{s}$ without
11. approx approximately
12. H_2O_2 hydrogen peroxide
13. L liters
14. sol solution
15. fld fluid
16. D&C dilation and curettage
17. pericare perineal care
18. $\overline{c}$ with
19. 1/2 one half
20. sm small
21. amt amount
22. vag vagina
23. hr hours

▶ Activity 3.12: Understanding Concise Wording

Complete Sentence	Thought Unit
1. ___h___ He is able to abduct right arm to shoulder height.	a. Full ROM (R) wrist and fingers
2. ___e___ He is unable to flex right elbow.	b. Warm, moist palms
3. ___a___ He has full range of motion in right wrist and fingers.	c. No BM
4. ___f___ Mr. A tells you that he took a long time to void and that he had pain while voiding.	d. 10 min duration
5. ___g___ He stated that he flushed urine down the toilet.	e. Unable to flex (R) elbow
6. ___d___ The pain lasted 10 minutes.	f. States that he voided with difficulty
7. ___c___ He has not moved his bowels.	g. Discarded urine by self
8. ___b___ The palms of her hands are warm and sweaty.	h. Able to abduct (R) arm to shoulder height
9. ___k___ Baby V took 2 ounces of Similac.	i. 30 mL clear fluid removed
10. ___m___ The baby was sleeping.	j. Legs in alignment
11. ___j___ Her hips, knees, and ankles are not turned–either outward or inward.	k. Similac–60 mL taken
12. ___o___ Mr. F–passes a lot of gas while he is expelling the enema.	l. Sm amt bleeding from vag
13. ___n___ Her respirations are below 16 breaths per minute.	m. Sleeping
14. ___i___ One ounce of clear fluid was removed through the needle.	n. Resp less than 16
15. ___l___ There is a small amount of blood coming from the vagina.	o. Expelling flatus

▶ Activity 3.13: Analyzing Effectiveness of Communication

1. Yes, the nurse is able to obtain information from Mr. Yang about his pain. She uses a series of questions that ask about various aspects of Mr. Yang's experience of pain. Because the questions were specific and focused on pain, Mr. Yang responded with information that will help the nurse assess and manage the pain.

2. The nurse begins with an open-ended question ("How are you doing?"), followed by a focused question ("Can you tell me more about how you are feeling right now?") and probes ("Are you in any pain right now?. . . Tell me more. Where is your pain?") to obtain information about Mr. Yang's experiences of pain. The most effective questions are those that ask about specific aspects of pain, such as location, intensity, quality, and duration. (See answers to Activity 3.14: Identifying Questions about Pain for a complete list of questions.)

3. Mr. Yang seems somewhat reluctant to talk about the pain he is currently experiencing or even to admit that he is experiencing pain. In response to the nurse's open-ended question at the beginning of the interview, he says, "I'm fine." However, because of the discrepancy between his verbal and nonverbal communication (he is breathing through clenched teeth), the nurse tests the discrepancy, "You say you're fine, but you seem to be in pain. Can you tell me more about how you are feeling right now?" Mr. Yang continues to downplay his pain, by responding, "I'm doing better than last night." The nurse's third question is more direct: "Are you in any pain right now?" to which Mr. Yang replies, "Yes, a little." With the third question, Mr. Yang finally answers the question even though he is still downplaying how much pain he is experiencing. (A little later, he rates his pain a 5 on a scale of 0 to 10, indicating moderate pain.) By asking questions that are increasingly more specific, the nurse is able to overcome Mr. Yang's reluctance to talk about the pain he is experiencing.

4. In some cultures, it may be a sign of weakness to admit that one is experiencing pain. With clients for whom this belief may be the case, nurses may need to first establish trust with the client. It may also be helpful to ask questions that are specifically about pain, as more specific questions focus on the facts, rather than feelings, the latter of which could provoke connotations of shame.

5. Overall, the nurse was effective in her response to the traditional remedies of cupping and pricking that Mr. Yang mentioned. She is not judgmental, but simply restates what Mr. Yang has said to make sure she has understood, "From what I hear you say, the traditional treatments of cupping and pricking provide some relief to the pain. Is that correct?" She also goes on to say that she is glad to hear that these treatments help him feel better. However, she could have asked a few follow-up questions about the traditional treatments, such as most recent treatment, frequency of treatment, and amount of relief obtained from treatment, as traditional medicine can interfere with the medical treatments Mr. Yang is receiving in the hospital. In addition, such questions validate the importance of clients being able to continue with traditional treatments that do not interfere with medical treatments, as they may be beneficial for clients for cultural and spiritual reasons.

▶ Activity 3.14: Identifying Questions about Pain

Aspect of Pain	Question from Dialog; Additional Question
Location	"Where is your pain?" "Can you tell me where you feel pain?"
Intensity	"On a scale of 0 to 10, with 0 no pain and 10 the worst pain you can imagine, how would you rate your pain?" "How bad is your pain?"
Radiating quality	"Tell me what your pain usually feels like." "What is your pain like?"
Movement	"Do you feel the chest pain radiating or moving to other parts of your body?" "Does the pain move elsewhere in your body?"
Time of onset	None. "When did (or does) the pain start?"
Duration	"How long does the pain usually last?" "How long have you had the pain?"
Constancy	None. "Does the pain ever go away?" ("When and for how long?")
Precipitating factors	"What triggers or causes the pain?" "What makes the pain worse?"
Alleviating factors	Two questions from dialog: "What relieves your pain or helps make it go away when you are at work?" "Is there anything else that helps to relieve your pain?" "What pain medications do you use?"
Associated symptoms	None. "Do you have any symptoms before, during, or after your pain, for example, nausea, dizziness, blurred vision, shortness of breath?"
Effects on activities of daily living (ADLs)	None. "How does the pain affect your daily life, for example, eating, sleeping, working, and social and recreational activities?"
Past pain experiences	None. "Tell me about your experiences with pain in the past."
Personal meaning of pain	"What do you fear most about your pain?" "What meaning do you give to your pain?"
Coping resources	None. "How do you cope with the pain?"
Affective response	None. "How does the pain make you feel—for example, anxious, depressed, frightened, tired, burdensome?"

▶ Activity 3.15: Understanding Client's Rating of Pain

Ratings of Pain:

Scenario #3: When Mr. Yang is first admitted to the hospital, he rates his pain at 8 out of 10, indicating "severe pain" on the traditional pain rating scale.

Dialog: During the interview with the nurse at the beginning of the day shift, Mr. Yang rates his pain at 5, indicating "moderate pain" on the traditional pain rating scale.

Progress Note: At the end of the day shift, Mr. Yang rates his pain at 2, indicating "mild pain" on the traditional pain rating scale.

Questions about Mr. Yang's Ratings of Pain:

1. The nurse interviews Mr. Yang about his pain at the beginning of the day shift. The night before, he had been given hydromorphone (Dilaudid) for pain relief. During the interview he rates his pain at a 5, indicating "moderate pain." So, although there has been a decrease in pain from the rating of 8 for "severe pain" the night before, Mr. Yang is still experiencing quite a bit of pain.
2. In some cultures, it may be a sign of weakness to admit that one is experiencing pain. With clients for whom this belief may be the case, nurses may need to first establish trust with the client. It may also be helpful to ask questions that are specifically about pain.
3. By the time of the progress note, Mr. Yang has had a myocardial infarction (heart attack). He has been on continuous IV morphine at 5 mg per hour for several hours, and he now rates his pain at 2, indicating "mild pain."

▶ Activity 3.16: Understanding Client's Descriptions of Pain

Mr. Yang uses the following adjectives in the dialog with the nurse to describe his pain: *killing, throbbing, burning, breathless, dizzy, stiff,* and *tight*. In Scenario #1, Mr. Yang describes his pain as *intense* and *radiating*.

Answers will vary. Listed are adjectives that are commonly used to describe pain. Some adjectives describe the sensory experience; others the affective experience. They are divided into levels of intensity of pain, as per the traditional pain rating scale (mild, moderate, severe, worst pain possible). Adjectives that refer to the pattern of pain (onset, duration, constancy of pain) are marked with (P).

Sensory Words

Mild	Moderate	Severe	Worst Pain Possible
diminishing (P)	chronic (P)	sudden (P)	crushing
intermittent (P)	constant (P)		piercing
receding (P)	continuous (P)	acute	scalding
sporadic (P)	persistent (P)	burning	searing
subsiding (P)	recurring (P)	cutting	stabbing
		deep	
mild	aching	drilling	
slight	blunt	electric	
sore	cold	gripping	
subtle	cramping	hammering	
tender	dull	heavy	
	hurting	hot	
	numb	intensifying	
	painful	jabbing	
	pressing	lightning	
	pricking	penetrating	
	stinging	pounding	
		pulsating	
		radiating	
		sharp	
		shooting	
		splitting	
		throbbing	
		wrenching	

Affective Words

Mild	Moderate	Severe	Worst Pain Possible
bearable	nagging (P)	debilitating	agonizing
manageable	gnawing (P)	exhausting	excruciating
not too bad		frightening	incapacitating
	annoying	intense	killing
	tiring	miserable	suffocating
	troublesome	punishing	terrifying
	uncomfortable	sickening	unbearable
		torturing	

▸ Activity 3.17: Identifying Open-Ended Questions

1. "How are you feeling?"	1. Open
2. "Are you feeling pain?"	2. Closed
3. "Tell me about the pain."	3. Open
4. "What are you doing for the pain?"	4. Open
5. "Are you taking any medication?"	5. Closed
6. "Are you available at 11 o'clock for your next appointment?"	6. Closed
7. "When are you available for your next appointment?"	7. Open
8. "Are you exercising regularly?"	8. Closed
9. "How often do you exercise?"	9. Closed
10. "Tell me about your physical activity."	10. Open

▸ Activity 3.18: Analyzing Dialog for Open-Ended Questions

At the beginning of the dialog, the nurse asks Mr. Yang: "How are you doing?" Mr. Yang responds, but does not reveal that he is feeling pain.

▸ Activity 3.19: Asking Open-Ended Questions

Nurse's Closed Question	Nurse's Open-Ended Alternative
1. "Where is the pain?"	1. "Tell me about the pain."
2. "Did you have a good week?"	2. "How have you been this week?"
3. "Do you have children?"	3. "Tell me about your family."
4. "You look sad. Are you depressed?"	4. "You look sad. How are you feeling?"
5. "Have you eaten today?"	5. "What have you been eating lately?"

▸ Activity 3.20: Analyzing Dialog for Focused Questions

After testing a discrepancy between Mr. Yang's verbal and nonverbal messages, the nurse asks a focused question: "Can you tell me more about how you are feeling right now?" Mr. Yang responds that he is doing better than earlier today, still not acknowledging that he is experiencing pain. The nurse then asks another focused question about Mr. Yang's pain: "... are you in any pain right now?" Mr. Yang responds: "Yes, a little," still downplaying his pain.

Note that the focused questions the nurse asks are closed. This may be because the nurse's initial open-ended question did not elicit a response from Mr. Yang.

▶ Activity 3.21: Asking Focused Questions

Nurse's Open-Ended Question	Nurse's Focused Question
1. "Tell me about the pain."	1. "Tell me about the pain in your leg."
2. "How have you been this week?"	2. "How have you been sleeping this week?"
3. "Tell me about your family."	3. "Do you have any children?"
4. "You look sad. How are you feeling?"	4. "Can you tell me about what happened this past week?"
5. "What have you been eating lately?"	5. "What did you have for breakfast today?"

▶ Activity 3.22: Analyzing Dialog for Probes

The nurse uses specific probes to ask Mr. Yang about various aspects of his pain:

"Where is your pain?"

"How would you rate your pain?"

"Tell me what your pain usually feels like."

"Do you feel the chest pain radiating or moving to other parts of your body?"

"How long does the pain last?"

"What triggers or causes the pain?"

"What relieves your pain or helps make it go away when you are at work?"

"Is there anything else that helps to relieve your pain?"

"What do you fear most about your pain?"

Mr. Yang seems more willing to respond to specific probes about his pain than to open-ended questions or focused questions.

▶ Activity 3.23: Analyzing Dialog for Paraphrasing

The nurse paraphrases twice to make sure the nurse has understood what Mr. Yang has said: "As I understand it, the pressure at work makes the pain worse and makes it harder for you to get your work done. Is that correct?" and "From what I hear you say, the traditional treatments of cupping and pricking provide some relief to the pain. Is that correct?" In both cases, Mr. Yang replies simply, "Yes." Paraphrasing thus helps to confirm the nurse's understanding of what Mr. Yang has said, but it does not seem to encourage him to add any additional information. Yet it may help to build trust between Mr. Yang and the nurse by showing him that the nurse cares and wants to understand his experience of pain.

▸ Activity 3.24: Paraphrasing

Client's Statement	Nurse's Paraphrase
1. "I haven't been sleeping well. I can't sleep at night and then I can't get up in the morning."	1a. Unacceptable: "Sounds like you're depressed." Reason why unacceptable: does not rephrase what client has said 1b. Acceptable: "You've been having trouble sleeping."
2. "The doctor told me to take 1 pill twice a day until the pills ran out, but I felt better the next day, so I stopped."	2a. Unacceptable: "You did not understand the doctor." Reason why unacceptable: expresses disapproval 2b. Acceptable: "You stopped taking the medication when you felt better even though your doctor told you to finish the prescription."
3. "I don't believe that smoking is bad for you. I've smoked a pack a day for 20 years."	3a. Unacceptable: "Maybe you'll believe that smoking is bad when you have a heart attack!" Reason why unacceptable: judging 3b. Acceptable: "You're not convinced that smoking is dangerous because it hasn't affected you."
4. "My child has a fever and sore throat. What should I do?"	4a. Unacceptable: "That sounds like a cold. Don't worry about it." Reason why unacceptable: cliché 4b. Acceptable: "You need some information about what to do for your child's fever and sore throat."
5. "I'd like to lose some weight, but the holidays are coming up."	5a. Unacceptable: "You should watch what you eat if you really want to lose weight." Reason why unacceptable: gives advice 5b. Acceptable: "You think this is a difficult time of year to lose weight."

▸ Activity 3.25: Analyzing Dialog for Clarification Requests

Mr. Yang trails off in the middle of a sentence and through his nonverbal communication indicates that his back is hurting. The nurse asks for clarification: "I'm sorry, I didn't understand the last part of what you said, but you seem to be uncomfortable. Could you repeat that?" In response, Mr. Yang states, "My back has been feeling stiff and tight." The clarification request is effective in getting Mr. Yang to talk about another kind of pain he has been experiencing.

▶ Activity 3.26: Analyzing Dialog for Discrepancy Tests

In response to the nurse's initial open-ended question, Mr. Yang says that he is fine, but at the same time he breathes through clenched teeth. The nurse follows up by testing the discrepancy between his verbal and non-verbal communication, "You say you're fine, but you seem to be in pain," followed by a focused question, "Can you tell me more about how you are feeling right now?" Mr. Yang responds with "I'm doing better than last night," but still seems to be downplaying the pain he is experiencing.

▶ Activity 3.27: Testing Discrepancies

Client's Discrepancy	Nurse's Response
1. A client is sitting in a clinic, waiting to be seen. The client seems preoccupied: He is wringing his hands and his eyes are watery. When asked how he feels, he says, "Just fine."	1. "You say you're just fine, but you seem preoccupied. How do you really feel?"
2. A client is grossly overweight. When asked about his diet, he claims that he does not eat much and always eats healthy food.	2. "You say you do not eat much and always eat healthy food. So, what do you think is causing you to be overweight?"
3. A client in the hospital says that her family visits regularly. Later, the client says she always feels lonely.	3. "You say you're always lonely. Before you told me that your family visits regularly. Can you tell me more about why you feel lonely?"
4. A client says that he does not smoke, yet his clothes smell of smoke and his teeth are heavily stained with nicotine.	4. "You told me that you do not smoke, yet your clothes smell of smoke. Can you explain why?"
5. You ask an elderly client what her address is, and the client responds, "1327 Marshall." Later, the client writes down "2713 Marshall."	5. "You told me your address is 1327 Marshall, but you wrote down that your address is 2713 Marshall. Do you remember which one is correct?"

▶ Activity 3.28: Analyzing Dialog for Summarizing

1. Toward the end of the interview, the nurse summarizes what Mr. Yang has said about his pain. The nurse begins with the following introductory sentence: "So, I would like to wrap up our conversation now, but before we finish, let me make sure that I have noted everything that you have said about your pain." Then she summarizes the interview: "Right now your pain is about a 5 on a scale of 0 to 10. Your pain is usually a throbbing, burning feeling in your chest that causes tightness, and sometimes the pain moves to your shoulder. More recently your back has been hurting, too. The pain in your chest usually lasts 10 minutes, but can last as long as 30 minutes. Getting overexerted in the restaurant seems to trigger the pain, but when you sit down and cool off, it gets better. Traditional treatments also seem to help. You also seem concerned about how the pain will affect your ability to work in the restaurant. Is there anything else you would like to add?"

2. In response to the nurse's question at the end of the summary, "Is there anything else you would like to add?" Mr. Yang replies: "Yes, I want to know what is wrong with me and what the doctors can do to help me get well." The summary seems to encourage Mr. Yang to ask a question about what he is most concerned about, indicating that a certain degree of trust has been established between the nurse and Mr. Yang.

   Without the introductory phrase and the request for confirmation, the summary would be less effective. An introductory phrase helps both the nurse and the client transition from asking and answering questions to reviewing the information that has been gathered. Without an introductory phrase, the client might not listen in the same way to make sure that everything that was important to the client was included in the summary. Without a request for confirmation, the client might not realize that the nurse had finished summarizing the interview. Furthermore, the client might not realize that the nurse wanted his or her input regarding whether all important points were included in the summary.

Activity 3.29: Summarizing

Case Notes	Summary
1. A pregnant client came to the clinic at 24 weeks for a prenatal visit. She is experiencing fatigue, edema, and abdominal pain. She expresses concern about her baby's health and her performance at work.	1. "From what you have said, you're concerned about your baby's health and your own performance at work. You've been having some issues with edema, abdominal pain and fatigue. Is that correct?"
2. A teenage female client came to the school nurse and was anxious because she almost fainted in class. She has been experiencing a burning sensation while urinating and often sweats uncontrollably. She has never felt this way before and her friends suggested that she go home for the day. She is worried about missing her final exam.	2. "As I understand, you've been sweating excessively and feel burning while urinating. In addition, you almost fainted. You have never felt this way before and you do not want to miss your final exam. Is that right?"
3. A male client diagnosed with a tibia fracture cannot feel his feet and fingers. He complains of drowsiness, thirst, and a severe headache. His wife and 2 children have not been in to see him and he is concerned about their well-being.	3. "You have a severe headache and are thirsty and drowsy. Your fingers and feet are numb and you are worried about your wife and children. Is there anything else?"

Activity 3.30: Opening and Closing an Interview

1. At the end of the dialog, after the nurse has summarized the conversation and Mr. Yang has had a chance to say something in response, the nurse closes by saying, "In the meantime, during my shift, I will do my best to make sure that your pain is controlled and that you feel comfortable and well-taken care of," a closing that also provides truthful reassurance. Mr. Yang says, "Thank you very much" and smiles, an indication that he is feeling more comfortable now.

2. One possibility would be: "Hello, my name is ______________________ and I'm a student nurse. I'll be on the floor until noon today. Would you mind if I ask you a few questions? It should take about 15 minutes or so."

3. "Thank you so much for your time. I've enjoyed talking with you. Just let me know if you need anything while I'm here. As I mentioned, I'll be on the floor until noon today."

4. If a client is likely to stay in the hospital for a while, it could be helpful to offer the possibility of continued interaction between the client and student nurse. It could help to create trust in the student nurse and confidence in the quality of health care that the client is receiving.

Activity 3.31: Considering Culture and Pain Management

Answers will vary.

Addressing Personal Health–Related Issues

4

Learning Objectives

- Addressing personal health–related issues
- Understanding language clients use to describe bodily functions
- Understanding medication orders
- Understanding medications and nursing actions
- Understanding the language of goals, desired outcomes, and nursing interventions
- Analyzing and evaluating documentation of client care
- Asking personal health–related questions
- Avoiding pitfalls to effective interviewing: Asking multiple questions, overusing closed questions, and asking "why" questions
- Recognizing cultural differences in exploring personal health–related issues

Scenario #4

Client: Hispanic* female, 17 yo

Diagnosis: Peptic ulcer disease

History: Bulimia nervosa (purging type), gastritis, asthma, intermittent GERD, pernicious anemia

Jamie Martínez is a 17-year-old adolescent whose parents immigrated to the United States from Mexico when she was 4. She was admitted to med/surg with a diagnosis of PUD (**peptic ulcer disease**). She has been vomiting blood for 2 days and has dark **tarry stools**. She is experiencing abdominal pain **flare ups**, especially at night due to increased gastric **secretions** and lying down. Her BP is 84/57 and her O_2 sats are 99%. She has a history of **bulimia nervosa (purging type), gastritis**, and **asthma.** For the past 2 years, she has had **intermittent bouts** of GERD (**gastroesophageal reflux disease**), which is managed with omeprazole. Her asthma is **dormant**; she has not had any asthma attacks in 6 years although she **wheezes** occasionally when her heartburn intensifies. During admission she stated, "I'm dying, my stomach is killing me, and my throat is on fire!" She rated her pain at 8 on a scale of 0 to 10. She is clearly anxious. Upon doing a health history, the **triage nurse** discovered that Jamie has had **pernicious anemia** for 2 years and, until recently, was on intensive vitamin B12 therapy to treat it. She is Full Code. She is allergic to codeine and latex. The attending physician ordered the following medications: 0.9% NS IV running at 100 mL/hr to maintain hydration and fluid balance; omeprazole 20 mg PO BID to reduce gastric acid **secretion**† ; famotidine 20 mg IV push BID to **inhibit** gastric acid secretion, to prevent acid-induced inflammation and promote healing of ulcer; amoxicillin 1,000 mg PO BID to **eradicate** bacteria causing the infection; hydrocodone/acetaminophen (Vicodin)‡ 10 mg PO q4–6hr PRN to relieve pain; and ibuprofen 400 mg PO PRN to reduce fever over 100.2°F. Her weight should be checked daily, and vital signs and O_2 sats checked q4h. If O_2 sats fall below 90%, the clinician should be contacted and O_2 at 2 L administered via NC to increase oxygenation. Pt should be encouraged to take **fluids orally**. After she has eaten, she should remain **upright** (either sitting in chair or at 90° in bed in a **high Fowler's position**) for 3 hours to decrease **acid reflux**, during which time vital signs should be monitored every 15 minutes because of hypotension. She is on a non-irritating diet. **Urine test** (or **urinalysis**) and CBC lab have been ordered. **Psychiatric** and dietician **consults** ordered. Jamie's parents are both professionals; they are very concerned about their daughter's well-being, but they are reluctant to acknowledge that she has an **eating disorder** and have not participated in any kind of family counseling. Her mother has been with her in the hospital since admission. The Martínez family is very involved in the Catholic church; their priest has visited every day since Jamie's admission. Jamie is a senior in high school and is on the honor roll and in the school orchestra.

**Hispanic* refers to citizens or residents of the United States who speak Spanish as their native or heritage language; *Latino* refers to peoples of Latin American origin or ancestry regardless of their language or ethnic background.

†gastric acid secretion = stomach acid

‡Vicodin is a combination of 2 generic medications: hydrocodone and acetaminophen.

Critical Thinking Skills: Addressing Personal Health–Related Issues

Addressing personal health–related issues such as sexuality, smoking cigarettes, drinking alcohol, and ingesting drugs is part of providing holistic care to clients. Yet both clients and nurses may be reluctant to discuss issues that are this personal. It is important for health care providers to consider the role of issues like this in a person's overall health and to practice strategies for addressing these issues in interviews with clients.

▶ Activity 4.1: Addressing Personal Health–Related Issues

Determine your answers to the following questions based on Scenario #4 about Ms. Martínez.

1. What type of personal health–related issue is Ms. Martínez experiencing? What are some of the physical as well as psychological issues associated with this illness?

   ____

   ____

2. What do you know about this type of illness? What do you think causes this illness? What do you think may have contributed to this illness for Ms. Martínez?

   ____

   ____

3. Why is a psychiatric consult ordered for Ms. Martínez? What might be some concerns that the parents have about a consultation with a psychiatrist?

   ____

   ____

4. What are some possible strategies to address this illness for Ms. Martínez, in particular strategies that reflect the nurse's awareness of and sensitivity toward culturally influenced beliefs, values, and practices?

   ____

   ____

Understanding and Using Language Effectively in Health Care Settings

The language used in health care settings is different from general, conversational English. Nurses must use medical/nursing terminology as well as specialized ways of communicating with clients. In addition, nurses must understand the language that clients use in the health care setting.

Client Talk: Describing Bodily Functions

The words that clients use to describe bodily functions and body parts are different from those that health care professionals use. To communicate effectively with clients, you need to understand the words clients use. You may also need to use some of these words in describing bodily functions so that your clients can understand you. If you are unsure whether a particular layperson's term is appropriate for a health care professional to use, ask a friend or colleague who is a native English speaker or an experienced nurse.

▶ Activity 4.2: Understanding Client Talk—Describing Bodily Functions

Match the layperson's term with the corresponding medical/nursing term. Write the letter of the medical/nursing term in the correct blank. The first one has been done for you.

Medical/Nursing Term(s)

a. cerumen
b. congestion
c. defecating
d. diaphoretic
e. diarrhea
f. emesis
g. epistaxis
h. eructation
i. flatulence
j. foul body odor
k. halitosis
l. pyrosis
m. mucus
n. nausea
o. perspiration
p. pulse
q. saliva
r. sinus drainage
s. urinating, voiding

Layperson's Term(s)

1. ____k____ bad breath
2. __________ snot
3. __________ spit
4. __________ bloody nose
5. __________ peeing
6. __________ heartbeat
7. __________ sweat
8. __________ feeling like you're going to vomit
9. __________ runny nose, post-nasal drip
10. __________ earwax
11. __________ stuffy nose
12. __________ pooping
13. __________ belching, burping
14. __________ the runs
15. __________ heartburn
16. __________ sweaty
17. __________ B.O., smelly
18. __________ farting, passing gas
19. __________ puke, barf, throw up, vomit

Medical/Nursing Vocabulary

How many of the bolded medical/nursing words used in Scenario #4 about Ms. Martínez do you already know? For those words you do not know, look them up in a nursing textbook, an English language medical dictionary, or online resources. Refer to the definitions in the Answer Key for Chapter Four, as needed.

Medical/Nursing Abbreviations

Identify as many of the abbreviations from Scenario #4 about Ms. Martínez as you can. Refer, as needed, to the list of Medical/Nursing Abbreviations in the Appendix.

Expansion of Medical/Nursing Abbreviations: Medication Orders

The medications that Ms. Martínez is currently taking are included in Scenario #4. Abbreviations and acronyms are commonly used in medication orders.

Medication Orders

There are 7 parts to a medication order. (See the Medication Orders section in Chapter One to review the 7 parts.) Chapter One talked about dose (part 4), Chapter Two discussed route of administration (part 5), and Chapter Three introduced frequency of administration (part 6). Here you will look at these 3 parts of medication orders together.

▶ Activity 4.3: Understanding Medication Orders

Write out the meaning of the following abbreviations. Use the lists in Chapters One, Two, and Three to help you.

1. tetracycline 250 mg PO QID ______________________
2. furosemide (Lasix) 40 mg PO stat ______________________
3. ampicillin 500 mg IV q6h ______________________
4. lente insulin 36 units subcut every a.m. AC ______________________
5. codeine 30 mg PO q4–6h PRN for pain ______________________
6. atorvastatin (Lipitor) 20 mg PO daily ______________________
7. insulin glargine (Lantus) 10 units subcut every a.m. ______________________
8. D_5W IV at 100 mL/hr ______________________
9. ceftriaxone (Rocephin) 500 mg IM ×1 ______________________
10. acetaminophen (Tylenol) 120 mg rectally q4h PRN T over 102° ______________________

Expansion of Scenario #4: Understanding Medications and Nursing Actions

When Ms. Martínez is admitted to the hospital, she is assessed by the attending physician, who orders medications, labs (laboratory tests), and other tests for her. In addition, both the physician and the nurse who is assigned to care for Ms. Martínez on the medical/surgical unit determine appropriate nursing actions. Some of these nursing care actions are carried out by the nurse, some by other health care professionals.

▶ Activity 4.4: Understanding Medications in Scenario #4

Match the purpose of each medication with its name. Write the letter of the purpose in the correct blank. Then, identify whether the route of each medication is PO (by mouth) or IV (intravenous).

Medication	Route	Purpose
1. __________ normal saline	__________	a. To reduce fever over 100.2°
2. __________ omeprazole	__________	b. To maintain hydration and fluid balance
3. __________ famotidine	__________	c. To eradicate bacteria causing the infection
4. __________ amoxicillin	__________	d. To relieve pain
5. __________ hydrocodone with acetaminophen	__________	e. To reduce gastric acid secretion
6. __________ ibuprofen	__________	f. To inhibit gastric acid secretion, prevent acid-induced inflammation, and promote healing of the ulcer

▶ Activity 4.5: Understanding Nursing Actions in Scenario #4

Match the purpose of each nursing action with the action. Write the letter of the purpose in the correct blank.

Nursing Action	Purpose
1. __________ maintain on non-irritating diet	a. To monitor vital signs, especially blood pressure, as client is hypotensive
2. __________ take daily weight	b. To replenish fluid loss from bleeding and dehydration
3. __________ take vitals every 4 hours	c. To decrease acid reflux after eating while assessing cardiovascular status
4. __________ check O_2 sats every 4 hours	d. To monitor for weight loss because of client's eating disorder
5. __________ contact clinician if O_2 sats fall below 90%	e. To treat peptic ulcer
6. __________ encourage fluids orally	f. To request new orders for client, as needed
7. __________ after eating, maintain client upright or elevate HOB at 90° for 3 hours and monitor vital signs every 15 minutes	g. To monitor for oxygen loss due to bleeding and dehydration

Expansion of Scenario #4: Plan of Care

When nursing students prepare for clinical, they often use forms like the Plan of Care (Figure 4-1) to record essential information about the client from the client's record and to plan for the client's care. Note that the route of medication is not always specified on the Plan of Care, as nurses would refer to the Medical Administration Record (MAR) before administering medications. This Plan of Care reflects care for Ms. Martínez during the day shift on her first day at the hospital. The vital signs recorded were taken at the beginning of the shift.

Figure 4-1: Plan of Care
Scenario #4

ROOM	DIET	OTHER	T / P / RR / BP
2970	Non-irritating	Full Code Contact precautions HOB in high Fowler's position for 3 hrs after meals Vicodin 10 mg q4–6 hr PRN	T 98.7, P 72, RR 15, BP 118/77
INITIALS	**ACTIVITY**		**O_2 sats** 99% RA†
JM			
Dx	**IVs**		**NOTES**
PUD	0.9% NS at 100 mL/hr Famotidine 20 mg push BID 0800 and 2000		If O_2 sats fall below 90%, contact clinician
MHx	**LABS/TESTS/APPTS**	**ASSESSMENTS**	
Bulimia nervosa (purging type) Gastritis Asthma Intermittent GERD Pernicious anemia	Urinalysis CBC Psychiatric consult Dietician consult	VS q4h (except PC* q 15 min for 3 hrs) O_2 sats q4h Daily weight	
MDs			
Dr. Zhang			
TREATMENTS			
O_2 at 2 L via NC if O_2 sats fall below 90%			
ALLERGY	**PAIN**		**OUTPUTS**
Codeine Latex	8/10		N/A

0700/1900	0800/2000 (circled)	0900/2100	1000/2200	1100/1300	1200/2400
	Omeprazole 20 mg Amoxicillin 1,000 mg				
1300/0100	**1400/0200**	**1500/0300**	**1600/0400**	**1700/0500**	**1800/0600**

*PC = after meals

†RA (room air) = regular conditions of breathing, without any added oxygen

▶ Activity 4.6: Plan of Care: Planning for Client's Care

Answer the following questions with information that is provided in the Plan of Care regarding Ms. Martínez.

1. What is Ms. Martínez's diagnosis?

   ____

   ____

2. What is Ms. Martínez's medical history?

   ____

   ____

3. What medication is Ms. Martínez given for pain? How much and how often?

   ____

   ____

4. What medications does Ms. Martínez receive twice daily? When is she given these medications, and how much of each medication does she receive?

   ____

   ____

5. What labs and appointments are planned for Ms. Martínez?

   ____

   ____

6. In what position is Ms. Martínez's HOB after meals? For how long?

   ____

   ____

Nursing Diagnosis: Addressing Ms. Martínez's Personal Health–Related Issues

Based on the information provided in the client's record and the nurse's assessment* of the client, the nurse writes a nursing diagnosis and a goal for treating the client. The nurse also identifies nursing interventions and desired outcomes to accomplish that goal. In planning holistic care for Ms. Martínez, the nurse identifies interventions that address her physiologic needs as well as her psychosocial needs with regard to her health-related issue. Review the interventions in Activity 4.7. Which nursing intervention reflects care of Mr. Martínez's psychosocial needs?

*A physical assessment is usually conducted when a client is first admitted to the hospital, either a head-to-toe assessment or a focused assessment on a specific problem area followed by a head-to-toe assessment, as needed. Information from this assessment is included in the client's record and is reviewed by the nurse caring for Ms. Martínez.

Nursing Diagnosis: Deficient fluid volume related to active fluid volume loss as manifested by dark tarry stools and decreased blood pressure.

Goal: Client will have adequate fluid volume.

▶ Activity 4.7: Nursing Diagnosis: Desired Outcomes and Nursing Interventions

Match each Desired Outcome for Ms. Martínez with the corresponding Nursing Intervention. Write the letter of the Desired Outcome in the correct blank.

Nursing Intervention	Desired Outcome
1. __________ Nurse will administer GI medication and analgesics and monitor for side effects during shift.	a. Blood pressure will be 120/80 mmHg by the end of shift.
2. __________ Nurse will monitor vital signs, lab values, and signs of GI bleeding closely throughout shift.	b. Hemoglobin and hematocrit will be within normal limits within 48 hours.
3. __________ Nurse will monitor fluid input and output closely throughout shift.	c. Client will describe expected daily dietary intake and adverse effects of purging by time of discharge.
4. __________ Nurse will teach client the importance of adequate nutritional intake and the consequences of purging by discharge date.	d. Client will report pain level of 3 (scale 0–10) and decreased anxiety within 1 hour of analgesic administration.

Expansion of Nursing Diagnosis: Understanding the Language of Goals, Desired Outcomes, and Nursing Interventions

Goals and Desired Outcomes for Clients

Once Nursing Diagnoses have been identified and prioritized, nurses and clients determine Goals and Desired Outcomes for each Nursing Diagnosis. Goals are the opposite of Nursing Diagnoses; that is, they represent healthy responses to the problem identified in the nursing diagnosis. For example, the goal *Improved nutritional status* is the opposite of the diagnosis *Imbalanced nutrition: Less than body requirements.* Likewise, the goal *Improved mobility* is the opposite of the diagnosis *Impaired physical mobility.*

Goals are stated broadly, whereas Desired Outcomes are specific, observable criteria that determine if the goals have been met. For the nursing diagnosis *Imbalanced nutrition: Less than body requirements*, the Goal is *Improved Nutritional Status.* If the client meets the Desired Outcome of *Gain[ing] 5 lb by April 25*, the client will achieve that goal.

Example #1:

Nursing Diagnosis	Goal (broad)	Desired Outcome (specific)
Imbalanced nutrition: Less than body requirements	Improved nutritional status	Gain 5 lb by April 25

Likewise, for the Nursing Diagnosis *Impaired physical mobility*, the Goals are *Improved mobility* and *Ability to bear weight on left leg*. If the client meets the Desired Outcomes of *Ambulate with crutches by end of week* and *Stand without assistance by end of month*, the client will achieve those goals.

Example #2:

Nursing Diagnosis	Goals (broad)	Desired Outcomes (specific)
Impaired physical mobility	Improved mobility	Ambulate with crutches by end of week
	Ability to bear weight on left leg	Stand without assistance by end of month

Connectors Used in Goals and Desired Outcomes

Goals and Desired Outcomes are sometimes combined into one statement, joined by *as evidenced by*.

Example:

Goal/Desired Outcome Improved nutritional status as evidenced by weight gain of 5 lb by April 25.

▶ Activity 4.8: Understanding Nursing Diagnoses and Goals

Match each Goal with the corresponding Nursing Diagnosis. Write the letter of the Goal in the correct blank.

Nursing Diagnosis	Goal
1. ________ Caregiver role strain	a. Express spiritual well-being
2. ________ Interrupted family processes	b. Improved communication
3. ________ Dysfunctional grieving	c. Healthy self-concept
4. ________ Impaired verbal communication	d. Experience control
5. ________ Ineffective coping	e. Diminished pain
6. ________ Disturbed body image	f. Improve family process
7. ________ Acute pain	g. Grieve appropriately
8. ________ Ineffective breastfeeding	h. Adequate role performance
9. ________ Readiness for enhanced spiritual well-being	i. Effective coping
10. ________ Powerlessness	j. Effective breastfeeding

▶ Activity 4.9: Matching Nursing Diagnoses and Goals

Match the Goals from Chapters One through Four with the corresponding Nursing Diagnosis. Write the letter of the Goal in the correct blank.

Nursing Diagnosis	Goal
1. __________ Impaired skin integrity	a. Adequate fluid volume
2. __________ Impaired spontaneous ventilation	b. Decrease in pain
3. __________ Acute pain	c. Improved skin integrity
4. __________ Deficient fluid volume	d. Adequate energy level and muscle function to maintain spontaneous breathing

Four Components of Desired Outcomes

In order for Desired Outcomes to be specific and observable, 4 language components are included.

1. **Subject:** The subject is usually the client or some part or attribute of the client. It is often omitted because it is understood. Sometimes the subject is the family.
2. **Action Verb:** The verb specifies what the client is to do—for example, *ambulate* and *stand.* They are observable behaviors. Verbs that are commonly used for writing Desired Outcomes are listed:

administer	demonstrate	move	sleep
ambulate	describe	perform	stand
apply	differentiate	rate	state
breathe	drink	recall	transfer
choose	explain	report	turn
consume	identify	show	use
define	list	sit	verbalize

3. **Conditions or Modifiers:** Conditions or modifiers specify *what* the action or behavior is or *how, when,* or *where* the patient will carry out the action or behavior.

   Examples:

   [will identify] *iron-rich foods* (what)

   with crutches (how) *by end of the week* (when)

   without assistance (how) *in the hospital* (where)

4. **Criteria of Desired Performance:** The criteria provide measurable indicators by which the patient's action or behavior will be evaluated, e.g., time *(how long* or *how often),* accuracy *(how well* or *how many),* distance *(how far),* and quality *(in what way).*

Examples:

Weighs 75 kg *by April* (time)

Lists *5 out of 6* signs of diabetes (accuracy)

Walks *1 block per day* (distance and time)

Administers insulin *using aseptic technique* (quality)

Avoid using words that are vague or that require interpretation. In the following examples, "increase daily exercise" and "improve knowledge of nutrition" are Desired Outcomes that are open to interpretation. Use specific, observable, measurable terms instead.

Examples:

Vague: Increase daily exercise

Specific: [Patient will] ambulate independently to nursing station back to room 3x/day by post-op day 2.

Vague: Improve knowledge of nutrition

Specific: [Client will] identify at least 3 sources of iron-rich foods prior to discharge from hospital.

▶ Activity 4.10: Understanding the Language of Desired Outcomes

Match the more specific wording with the vague wording for each of the Desired Outcomes. Write the letter of the specific wording in the correct blank.

Desired Outcomes–Vague Wording	Desired Outcomes–Specific Wording
1. __________ less pain	a. will report absence of nausea throughout day shift
2. __________ feel rested	b. will use 2 or fewer ABD dressings to incision site per 8-hour shift
3. __________ understand better	c. will have urine output of at least 30 mL/hr for 8-hour period
4. __________ less nausea	d. will attend all therapy sessions
5. __________ adequate voiding	e. will verbalize understanding of discharge instructions
6. __________ less anxious	f. will identify at least 3 factors that can be controlled by client
7. __________ less drainage	g. will demonstrate one or more relaxation techniques before invasive procedure
8. __________ increased appetite	h. will rate pain 3 or less on scale of 0–10
9. __________ experience increased sense of control	i. will consume at least 70% of all meals
10. __________ participate in activities	j. will have at least 4 hours of uninterrupted sleep at night

Analyzing the Language of Nursing Interventions

When Goals and Desired Outcomes have been determined, nursing interventions are then selected that will result in reducing or eliminating the etiology of the nursing diagnosis. Interventions are written in the nursing care plan as Nursing Interventions or actions that the nurse performs to help the client achieve his or her goals.

Three Components of Nursing Interventions

Nursing Interventions include 3 language components:

1. **Action Verb:** The verb states the order in a precise way (for example, *explain* instead of "teach"). It must be specific (for example, *the actions of insulin* instead of "insulin") and, whenever possible, *measurable* (for example, *measure and record* instead of "assess"). Note that "the nurse will" and "the client" are not written out, as they are understood.

    General: [The nurse will] teach [the client] about insulin

    Specific: *Explain* the actions of insulin

    General: Assess edema of left ankle daily

    Specific: *Measure and record* ankle circumference daily at 0900

    General: Put spiral bandage on left leg

    Specific: *Apply* spiral bandage *firmly* to left lower leg

2. **Content Area:** The content specifies the "what" and "where" of the order. In the example, *Apply spiral bandage firmly to left lower leg*, "spiral bandage" specifies *what* and "left lower leg" specifies *where.*
3. **Time Element:** The time element specifies "when," "how long," or "how often" the nursing order is to occur. In the example, *Measure and record ankle circumference at 0900 daily*, "at 0900" specifies *when* and "daily" specifies *how often.*

▶ Activity 4.11: Understanding Nursing Interventions

For each of the Nursing Interventions, circle the verb, underline once the Content Area ("what" and "where"), and underline twice the Time Element ("when," "how long," and "how often"). The first one has been done for you.

1. Monitor for verbalization of help needed to use commode after every meal.
2. Instruct patient to avoid drinking alcohol while on medication.
3. Raise the head of bed during periods of shortness of breath.
4. Discuss with client and spouse cancer support group resources before discharge.
5. Palpate abdomen for tenderness once during the shift.
6. Teach Kegel exercises to prevent urinary incontinence while sneezing, coughing, or laughing before end of shift.

7. Demonstrate blood pressure assessment technique once and repeat as needed.

8. Monitor blood glucose testing skills every shift.

9. Assess newly inserted gastric tube site for S/S (signs and symptoms) of infection every 8 hours.

10. Reposition patient every 2 hours.

Telephone Report

Nurses sometimes contact the clinician about a client by telephone, for example, when there is a medical emergency or when there is a significant or noteworthy change in the client's condition.

The nurse caring for Ms. Martínez contacts the attending physician by telephone about a change in Ms. Martínez's condition. Here is what the nurse reports to the physician, referred to as a *telephone report*:

> *Hello, Dr. Zhang. This is Sirri Ayawo, the RN caring for Ms. Jamie Martínez, a 17-year-old girl, in Room 2970. She was diagnosed with PUD and is experiencing intense burning in her stomach and esophagus. She has a history of bulimia nervosa, gastritis, asthma, intermittent GERD, and pernicious anemia. She has a 0.9% normal saline IV running at 100 milliliters per hour. She ate a few bites of her meal, and then I found her kneeling over the toilet vomiting. She just vomited 650 milliliters of bloody vomitus and is wheezing. About 30 minutes ago, she had a bowel movement and her stool was dark and tarry. Her gastric pH* is 2; she is complaining of intense stomach pain again and is quite weak and pale. Her O_2 sats are currently at 92% and her BP is 97/60. Her bowel sounds are hyperactive[†] in the left and right upper quadrants.[‡] I suspect that she continues to have gastric hemorrhaging[§] that is keeping her hypotensive[#] and dehydrated, and based on her CBC values, possibly anemic.[¶] How would you like us to proceed with her care?*

*pH measures the acidity or alkalinity of a solution. The pH scale ranges from 0 to 14 and measures how acidic or alkaline a substance is. A pH of 7 is neutral. A pH less than 7 is acidic. A pH greater than 7 is alkaline. A gastric pH of 2 is very acidic.

[†]hyperactive = abnormal bowel sounds, characterized by high-pitched, loud, rushing sounds that occur frequently, such as every 2–3 seconds

[‡]quadrant = 1 of 4 areas of the abdomen that is used to locate and describe abdominal findings

[§]hemorrhaging = bleeding

[#]hypotensive = suffering from low blood pressure

[¶]anemic = condition in which the number of red blood cells or the quantity or quality of hemoglobin is decreased

▶ Activity 4.12: Understanding Telephone Report

Review the telephone report about Ms. Martínez and compare with Scenario #4 and the Plan of Care. Answer the following questions.

1. In Scenario #4, the nurse reports that Ms. Martínez has been vomiting blood for 2 days. In the telephone report, she has just vomited. In what ways are these 2 instances of vomiting similar and different?

____

____

____

2. In Scenario #4 and in the telephone report, the nurse reports that Ms. Martínez's stool is dark and tarry. Why is her stool dark and tarry?

____

____

3. In Scenario #4, Ms. Martínez's O_2 sats are reported as 99%. In the telephone report, they are reported as 92%. Why have her O_2 sats dropped?

____

____

4. In Scenario #4, Ms. Martínez's blood pressure is reported as 84/57 mm Hg, which is hypotensive or low. In the Plan of Care, the BP is within normal range (118/77 mm Hg), but in the telephone report, it is again low (97/60 mm Hg). Why does Ms. Martínez's BP initially increase and then decrease?

____

____

____

Documentation of Telephone Report

After completing the telephone report, the nurse documents the date, the time, the person called, the person who received the information, what information was given, and what information was received. Figure 4-2 shows the documentation of the telephone report about Ms. Martínez.

Figure 4-2: Documentation of Telephone Report

> 10-27-13 1830 Jamie Martínez. Bloody vomitus and wheezing. Dark tarry stools. Severe stomach pain, weak and pale. Hyperactive bowel sounds in upper Ⓛ and Ⓡ quadrants.* O_2 sats 92%. Decreased BP and dehydration. Dr. Zhang notified via phone.---------------------------------S. Ayawo, RN

*In spoken language, the term "left and right upper quadrants" is used; in written language, "upper Ⓛ and Ⓡ quadrants" is used.

Telephone Order

In response to telephone reports, clinicians usually change medication and other orders for the client. Here is the attending physician's response to the nurse's report about Ms. Martínez, referred to as a *telephone order* (T.O.). Note that spoken delivery of medication orders differs in some ways from written orders.

> *Hello, Sirri. From your brief summary of Ms. Martínez in Room 2970, she is experiencing an increase in gastric acid which is causing the ulcers to bleed. Administer 80 milligrams of esomeprazole (Nexium) PO once immediately to reduce the acid reflux.* Administer 325 milligrams of ferrous sulfate PO once daily to boost her iron especially now with the hemorrhaging, and administer 10 milligrams of hydrocodone with acetaminophen PO every 4 hours to control her pain. Increase 0.9% normal saline IV to 150 milliliters per hour to increase her fluid volume. Administer 2 puffs of albuterol inhaler PRN every 4 to 6 hours to control the wheezing. Administer 2 liters of oxygen until her O_2 sats increase to 97% on room air. Collect sample of her vomitus and stool and send to the lab for testing and analysis. Also, order another CBC lab. Monitor BP every 15 minutes for 12 hours because of bleeding and drop in blood pressure, and encourage lots of clear fluid. I will see her in about 20 minutes when I am done with the client in my office. Thank you.*

*Heartburn

Documentation of Telephone Order

The nurse must document telephone orders from the physician. Figure 4-3 shows the nurse's documentation of the telephone order about Ms. Martínez, referred to as a *telephone order report.*

Figure 4-3: Telephone Order Report

1. Administer esomeprazole 80 mg PO once stat
2. Administer ferrous sulfate 325 mg PO once daily
3. Administer hydrocodone with acetaminophen 10 mg PO q4h
4. Increase 0.9% NS IV to 150 mL/hr
5. Administer albuterol inhaler 2 puffs PRN q4–6hr
6. Administer O_2 at 2 L until O_2 sats greater than 97% on RA
7. Collect vomitus sample
8. Collect stool sample
9. Order another CBC lab
10. Monitor BP q15 min for 12 hrs
11. Encourage lots of flds

10-27-13 1845

T.O. from Dr. Zhang /Sirri Ayawo, RN

Activity 4.13: Understanding Telephone Order

Answer the following questions based on the telephone order report about Ms. Martínez.

1. What new medication is Ms. Martínez given once daily? Why? In what form is this medication given?

____

____

2. How much hydrocodone with acetaminophen (Vicodin) is ordered for Ms. Martínez? In Scenario #4, how much hydrocodone with acetaminophen was she given? Is there a difference in the amount of medication? Are there other differences in the 2 medication orders for hydrocodone with acetaminophen? If so, what are they and why?

____

____

____

3. Which medication is Ms. Martínez given immediately? How much? How often?

____

____

4. How often is Ms. Martínez given albuterol? Why? How is the albuterol given? How much is given?

____

____

5. How much normal saline is ordered for Ms. Martínez in the telephone order? In Scenario #4, how much normal saline was ordered? Why is there a difference in the amount of medication?

____

____

____

6. How often is Ms. Martínez's blood pressure checked? In Scenario #4, how often was it checked? Why is there a difference in the frequency?

____

____

____

Documentation of Client Care: Progress Note

At the end of the shift, the nurse documents the care that was given to the client in the form of a progress note. Here is the progress note about the care that was provided to Ms. Martínez.

Progress Note

Identify Problem(s)

Bleeding ulcers, severe stomach and throat pain, decreased blood pressure, dehydration, decreased food intake, purging, and disturbed body image

Desired Outcome(s)

Pt will have decreased bleeding from the ulcers within 48 hours of treatment.

Pt will have increased comfort in stomach and throat within 24 hours of treatment.

Pt will have stabilized blood pressure within 12 hours.

Pt will maintain normal fluid balance within 24 hours of treatment.

Pt will have increased nutritional intake within 48 hours of treatment.

Pt will have decreased purging by the end of shift.

Pt will have improved body image within 48 hours of treatment and therapy.

Evaluation

VSS except BP 97/70. MD notified of BP; he increased 0.9% NS IV to 150 mL/hr to increase BP and fluid volume. Pt c/o of severe pain in her throat and stomach. MD notified; MD ordered hydrocodone with acetaminophen 10 mg PO q4h. 1st dose already administered at 1515; 2nd dose due in 4 hours, at 1915. Pt on non-irritating diet and eats 50% of meals. Pt's HOB upright for 3 hours after meals, to decrease acid reflux, during which time vitals taken every 15 minutes to assess cardiovascular status. Pt has nausea and vomited bloody vomitus after a few bites of her meal and her bowel sounds are active. Pt received O_2 at 2 L via NC and was wheezing during unstable period. Pt taking 2 puffs of albuterol inhaler PRN q4–6 hr to control wheezing. During periods of wheezing, pt is slightly nervous and needs reassurance when inhaler is administered. Her weight needs to be measured daily and changes reported to MD and dietician. Pt encouraged to use incentive spirometer q2h. Her parents and priest are supportive.

Plan

Continue to monitor client health status and progress. Continue to administer medications per MAR. Teach pt importance of keeping HOB upright 3 hours after meals, and drinking lots of fluids. Encourage pt to eat progressively more food as tolerated and to avoid purging. Pt willing to meet with eating disorder therapist. Provide quiet, healing environment for pt to promote well-being. Discuss plan of care with pt and family. Encourage pt to inform nurse of any concerns regarding her health and care.

▶ Activity 4.14: Addressing Personal Health–Related Issues

Determine your answers to the following questions based on the care provided to Ms. Martínez.

1. At the beginning of the shift, the nurse plans care for Ms. Martínez based on 4 nursing interventions (see Nursing Diagnosis: Addressing Ms. Martínez's Personal Health–Related Issues). How does each of the nursing interventions address the client's eating disorder? In what ways do these nursing interventions reflect holistic care of the client?

    ____

    ____

    ____

    ____

2. In the evaluation of the client in the progress note, the nurse refers to the "unstable period." What happened during the unstable period? (Review Telephone Report, as needed.)

    ____

    ____

    ____

3. What aspects of the plan (of care) in the progress note address the client's eating disorder? How does this plan reflect holistic care of the client?

    ____

    ____

    ____

    ____

4. In what ways does the plan (of care) in the progress note represent culturally competent care of the client's eating disorder? In what other ways could the nurse provide culturally competent care for the client's eating disorder?

    ____

    ____

    ____

    ____

Expansion of Documentation of Client Care: Analyzing and Evaluating Documentation

In Chapters One through Three, you were introduced to characteristics of effective documentation. Review this information in preparation for analyzing and evaluating an example of documentation of client care.

▶ Activity 4.15: Analyzing and Evaluating Documentation

Read the information about Mrs. Parker and the documentation that follows. Analyze and evaluate the documentation based on the characteristics of effective documentation discussed in Chapters One through Three, such as correct formatting, conciseness, objectivity, completeness, and preciseness. Answer the questions that follow.

> Mrs. Parker, a 67-year-old female, is admitted for knee pain. She has a past medical history of arthritis and osteoporosis. She told the admitting nurse that she can no longer do as much physically because of chronic pain and stiffness.
>
> 10 – Client is a worrier. I talked with her for a while with no success. She complains of pain in her knees.
>
> BP 128/87 130/90 P 75 RR 16
>
> 11 – Refused to take a bath.
>
> 12 – Client fell in the bathroom.

1. What guidelines were *not* followed in this documentation? Evaluate the documentation in terms of its formatting, conciseness, objectivity, completeness, and precision.

____

____

____

____

____

____

____

____

____

____

2. The nursing diagnosis for Mrs. Parker is *Impaired physical mobility related to stiffness*. What should the nurse include in the documentation?

____

____

____

____

Use the following statements to answer questions 3–6:

a. "I couldn't sleep at all last night"

b. Positioned supine with pillow behind head

c. Muscle relaxant relieves stiffness in knees

d. Pt rated pain at 6 on a scale of 0 to 10

e. "I can move my knees more easily now" (after interventions)

f. Muscle relaxant administered 2 hours ago

g. Warm pack placed around knees

h. BP 128/87 P 75 RR 16

i. Give muscle relaxant around the clock q6h

j. "Dull, constant pain in knees that radiates to thighs"

k. Rubs knees constantly

l. Pt rated pain at 3 on a scale of 0 to 10 after interventions

m. Perform passive ROM exercises to legs, as tolerated

3. Which statement(s) represent subjective data? ____________________

4. Which statement(s) represent objective data? ____________________

5. Which statement(s) represent nursing actions and interventions? ____________________

6. Which statement(s) represent outcomes? ____________________

Communication Skills: Pitfalls to Interviewing

In Chapter Three, you were introduced to interviewing techniques that are used to gather information from a client. However, just like with blocks to therapeutic communication (Chapter Two), there are pitfalls to effective interviewing. Read the dialog between the nurse and Ms. Martínez. Notice the various ways in which the nurse prevents the effective use of interviewing techniques with the client.

Dialog between Nurse and Ms. Martínez

Nurse: Good afternoon, Ms. Martínez.

Ms. Martínez: Hi. (looking disinterested)

Nurse: I know the past week has been quite challenging for you healthwise and a lot has been going on. What have you been eating this past month? How much do you eat at one time? How often do you eat?

Ms. Martínez: Well, sometimes I don't want to eat, and other times I want to eat a lot.

Nurse: What do you like eating?

Ms. Martínez: Mostly pizza, muffins, sweet potato fries, hamburger, and chicken tenders.

Nurse: Why do you eat these foods?

Ms. Martínez: What do you mean . . . ? I just like to eat them! (rising intonation and a negative tone in her voice)

<u>Nurse</u>: *Oh, I didn't mean it in a negative way. How often do you eat these foods?*

<u>Ms. Martínez</u>: *Anytime I want to.*

<u>Nurse</u>: *Are there certain situations in which you eat more or less food?*

<u>Ms. Martínez</u>: *Not really, I just stuff myself and then . . . . (looks away)*

<u>Nurse</u>: *And then what?*

<u>Ms. Martínez</u>: *(remains silent)*

<u>Nurse</u>: *Why won't you tell me? I care about your well-being.*

<u>Ms. Martínez</u>: *Because people will judge me, and I kind of feel that way right now.*

<u>Nurse</u>: *I'm very sorry for making you feel that way. (pause) How do you feel about your health?*

<u>Ms. Martínez</u>: *I'm just so tired of all these health problems. I caused these ulcers and I hate myself for it! (voice quivering)*

<u>Nurse</u>: *Don't blame yourself. What makes you think you caused it?*

<u>Ms. Martínez</u>: *I make myself throw up after eating a lot; so much of what I eat is nasty anyway. And then I have all this burning in my throat and stomach. I just want to . . . be . . . normal . . . a-a-again.. (crying)*

<u>Nurse</u>: *Why do you make yourself vomit after you eat?*

<u>Ms. Martínez</u>: *I don't know. (looks away)*

<u>Nurse</u>: *Do you have friends at school?*

<u>Ms. Martínez</u>: *A few. (looks away, eyes begin to water)*

<u>Nurse</u>: *Are you dating anyone?*

<u>Ms. Martínez</u>: *(shakes head) No.*

<u>Nurse</u>: *Do you drink alcohol or take drugs?*

<u>Ms. Martínez</u>: *(shakes head) A lot of kids at my school do, but I'm not interested in that.*

<u>Nurse</u>: *Do you have a good relationship with your parents?*

<u>Ms. Martínez</u>: *It's okay. (looks down)*

<u>Nurse</u>: *Tell me about school.*

<u>Ms. Martínez</u>: *What do you mean?*

<u>Nurse</u>: *Are you happy in your school?*

<u>Ms. Martínez</u>: *Not really. (quietly)*

<u>Nurse</u>: *Tell me more.*

<u>Ms. Martínez</u>: I feel so alone most of the time. (voice breaking) I'm the only, you know, brown person in my class. We live in the suburbs, and it's mostly white kids. My parents want me to get good grades and be a doctor, but they don't understand. No one even notices me in school. I'm quiet in class, and the teachers don't even know my name. They never call on me. (voice rising and talking quickly) The students just ignore me. I'm not popular and I don't wear designer clothes. I'm not tall and thin like they are; I'm short and overweight, and I have black hair, not blond hair. Every day my parents remind me how much they sacrificed coming to this country. They tell me they want me to be a doctor, but they never ask me what I want. I hate my life. (pause) I feel so much pressure to be someone I'm not. (pause) I just want to be like everyone else.

<u>Nurse</u>: Would you like to talk with a therapist about some of these issues? I'm particularly concerned about your bulimia and its effects on your health. We have a therapist on staff who specializes in working with young people with eating disorders. She can help you understand what you are going through and suggest more positive ways of dealing with the stresses of growing up, so you can be healthy again and stay healthy.

<u>Ms. Martínez</u>: Yes, I think I would like that. But, do my parents have to know?

<u>Nurse</u>: We can provide some services to adolescents without informing their clients, including seeing a therapist. At some point, you may decide to tell your parents, but we will keep that information confidential. How does that sound?

<u>Ms. Martínez</u>: Okay.

<u>Nurse</u>: I will make the referral right now. Perhaps the therapist can see you later today or tomorrow. I will let you know.

<u>Ms. Martínez</u>: Thank you.

<u>Nurse</u>: Let me know if there is anything else I can do for you.

<u>Ms. Martínez</u>: Okay. Thanks.

▶ Activity 4.16: Analyzing Effectiveness of Communication

Determine your answers to the following questions about the ineffectiveness of the nurse's communication with Ms. Martínez in the dialog.

1. What are some examples of the nurse's ineffective communication with Ms. Martínez?

____

____

____

2. What is the effect of the nurse's ineffective communication on Ms. Martínez?

____

____

____

3. Is the nurse able to gather information about Ms. Martínez's eating disorder? Why or why not?

____

____

____

4. Is the interview an example of therapeutic communication between the nurse and Ms. Martínez? Why or why not?

____

____

____

5. How could the nurse be more effective in her communication with Ms. Martínez?

____

____

____

6. Do you think the nurse is obligated to inform Ms. Martínez's parents that their daughter will be seeing a therapist? Why or why not?

____

____

____

Expansion of Dialog: Asking Personal Health–Related Questions

An essential part of any interview of a client is asking about personal health–related issues, such as sexual functioning, alcohol and drug use, and smoking. These questions can be difficult for a nurse to ask, and they can also be difficult for a client to answer.

To put the client at ease and to help create an atmosphere of trust, nonverbal communication is just as important as the questions themselves. Nurses must convey through their manner—specifically their posture, facial expression, tone of voice, rate of breathing, and rate of speech—a message of unconditional acceptance of anything the client says or does in response to these questions.

Once an atmosphere of trust and acceptance has been established, the specific skills used to ask about personal health–related topics are the same as talking about any other topic. For example, open-ended questions or focused questions can be used to begin this part of the interview, followed by probes, requests for clarification, and summation. In addition, therapeutic communication skills, such as verbal and nonverbal reassurance and reflection, may also be useful, as clients are unlikely to be comfortable discussing these topics.

The following are examples of questions that can be useful in initiating a discussion of personal health–related issues. Most of these questions are closed focused questions; however, follow-up questions can also be open-ended probes, for example, the follow-up question to the adolescent about sex.

Sex (to an adolescent): Do you have a boyfriend/girlfriend? How do you spend your time together?

Sex (to an adult): Are you in a significant relationship? Are you and your (partner, wife, husband) sexually active?

Drinking: Do you drink alcohol?

Drugs: Do you use any street drugs?

Smoking: Do you smoke?

After any of these initial questions or lead-ins, the nurse should watch and listen carefully to the client's response. The nature of the client's response will indicate how the interview should proceed: with focused questions and probes to obtain more information; with reflection and verbal/nonverbal reassurance to convey empathy and active listening; or with a temporary change of topic. It is important not to change the topic inappropriately just because the nurse is uncomfortable. However, if the topic seems to be uncomfortable for the client, it would be appropriate for the nurse to openly acknowledge the discomfort and suggest that they talk about the topic at a later time. For example, the nurse could say: *"I see this is an uncomfortable topic for you. Should we talk about it later?"*

▶ Activity 4.17: Analyzing Dialog for Personal Questions

Look back at the dialog between the nurse and Ms. Martínez. Identify any examples of personal questions that the nurse asks Ms. Martínez. Is the nurse able to obtain information about personal health–related issues from Ms. Martínez?

____

____

____

____

____

____

Expansion of Dialog: Pitfalls to Effective Interviewing (Asking Multiple Questions, Overusing Closed Questions, and Asking "Why" Questions)

In gathering information from a client, there are pitfalls for the nurse to avoid, as they can prevent or hinder an effective interview. Some of these pitfalls are asking multiple questions, overusing closed questions, and asking "why" questions.

Asking Multiple Questions

Multiple questions are a series of questions presented to the client one right after the other, without a pause in between. They are confusing to the client because it is not clear which one should be answered first. Also, the client could forget one of the questions and become anxious about having forgotten what was asked, rather than focusing on his or her answer.

Examples:

"Where do you live, in an apartment or house, and what is your neighborhood like?"

"Did you forget the appointment, or did you have something else, or did you call and the line was busy?"

Multiple questions should be broken down into separate questions. The nurse should pause between questions and wait for the client to respond.

"Where do you live?" (pause)

"Do you live in an apartment or house?" (pause)

"What is your neighborhood like?" (pause)

Another option is asking one broad open-ended question:

"Tell me about your neighborhood."

Sometimes, a nurse will ask one question and, if the client does not immediately answer, the nurse will ask another question, assuming the client did not understand the first. The nurse should give the client enough time to answer each question one at a time. If the client has not understood the first question, the nurse should rephrase that same question, rather than going on to another one.

▶ Activity 4.18: Analyzing Dialog for Multiple Questions

Look back at the dialog between the nurse and Ms. Martínez. Identify any examples of multiple questions that the nurse asks Ms. Martínez. What effect does the use of multiple questions have on Ms. Martínez?

____

____

____

____

▶ Activity 4.19: Transforming Multiple Questions

Practice asking one question at a time of the client. Transform each of the multiple questions on the left into a series of single questions or one broad open-ended question. The first one has been done for you.

Multiple Questions	Transformation
1. "How do you feel this morning–did you get enough sleep last night and enough to eat for breakfast?"	1. "How do you feel this morning?" (pause for reply) "How did you sleep last night?" (pause for reply) "How was breakfast?" (pause for reply)
2. "Where do you live, how many people live with you, and who do you live with?"	2. ____________________ ____________________
3. "Did stress, diet, exercise, or something else cause the problem?"	3. ____________________ ____________________

Note that for Transformation #1, open-ended questions have been asked instead of closed questions. For example, *"How did you sleep last night?"* replaces "Did you get enough sleep last night?" and *"How was breakfast?"* replaces "[Did you get] enough to eat for breakfast?" Open-ended questions are preferable to closed questions at the beginning of an interview because they encourage clients to talk.

▶ Activity 4.20: Practice Avoiding Multiple Questions

Review the dialog between the nurse and Ms. Martínez. Write down the examples of multiple questions that you identified. What questions could the nurse have used instead? Write alternative questions that the nurse could have used.

Examples of Multiple Questions	Alternative Questions
______________________	______________________
______________________	______________________
______________________	______________________
______________________	______________________
______________________	______________________

Overusing Closed Questions

In contrast to open-ended questions, closed questions can be answered with just 1 or 2 words (often just yes or no). Obviously there are situations when closed questions are preferable, such as when specific information is needed. However, closed questions can be overused, especially when the purpose of the question is to open up a new area of inquiry or to probe an unexplored topic of concern.

The following interview with a client is ineffective because of the nurse's overuse of closed questions. Note the effect that the overuse of closed questions has on the client by the end of the interview.

Nurse: "Do you take any medication for your pain?"

Client: "Yes."

Nurse: "Do you take prescription medications?"

Client: "Yes."

Nurse: "Do massages help?"

Client: "A little."

Nurse: "Does heat give you any relief?"

Client: "Sometimes."

Nurse: "Is there anything else you do for your pain?"

Client: "Yes." (Frowns)

Nurse: "What is it?"

Client: "Do you want to know what I do?"

Because of the nurse's overuse of closed questions, the interview becomes an interrogation with the nurse doing most of the talking. The barrage of questions puts the client on the defensive and discourages the client from talking. More effective than a series of closed questions would be an open-ended question, such as "*Tell me what you do for your pain,*" followed by appropriate focused questions and closed probes.

Sometimes, a series of closed questions is appropriate, such as with a checklist of items to be asked. The effect of such questioning can be mitigated, however, with an introductory comment:

"*Now I need to ask you a series of questions. Just answer with a simple 'yes/no' response for now.*"

▶ Activity 4.21: Analyzing Dialog for Closed Questions

Look back at the dialog between the nurse and Ms. Martínez. Identify any examples of the overuse of closed questions that the nurse asks Ms. Martínez. What effect does the overuse of closed questions have on Ms. Martínez?

____

____

____

____

____

▶ Activity 4.22: Transforming Closed Questions

Practice asking open-ended questions of the client. Rewrite the closed questions on the left so they are open-ended. The first one has been done for you.

Closed Questions	**Open-Ended Questions**
1. "Are you feeling pain?"	1. "Tell me about the pain."
2. "Are you taking any medication?"	2. ______________________________
3. "Are you available at 11 o'clock for your next appointment?"	3. ______________________________
4. "Are you exercising regularly?"	4. ______________________________
5. "How often do you exercise?"	5. ______________________________

▶ Activity 4.23 Practice Avoiding Closed Questions

Review the dialog between the nurse and Ms. Martínez. Write down the examples of closed questions that you identified. What questions could the nurse have used instead? Write alternative questions that the nurse could have used.

Examples of Closed Questions	Alternative Questions
______________________	______________________
______________________	______________________
______________________	______________________
______________________	______________________

Asking "Why" Questions

Another pitfall to effective interviewing is the use of "why" questions. They imply that clients should have an immediate explanation for their behavior or feelings and that something is wrong if a client does not.

Examples:

"Why do you smoke?"

"Why are you sad?"

"Why didn't you complete your exercises?"

"Why" questions should be rephrased to avoid the perception of disapproval, as well as to more accurately reflect what the nurse is asking for. In the first question "Why do you smoke?" the nurse may really want to know what the client understands about the dangers of smoking. A more accurate question would be: "*What concerns do you have about smoking?*" or "*Tell me what you know about the dangers of smoking.*"

The second question "Why are you sad?" could be rephrased as a request, "*Tell me what you are feeling.*" And the third question "Why didn't you complete your exercises?" could be rephrased as, "*How was the exercising?*" or "*I noticed you didn't complete your exercises. What happened?*"

▶ Activity 4.24: Analyzing Dialog for "Why" Questions

Look back at the dialog between the nurse and Ms. Martínez. Identify any examples of "why" questions that the nurse asks Ms. Martínez. What effect does the use of "why" questions have on Ms. Martínez?

____

____

____

____

____

▶ Activity 4.25: Transforming "Why" Questions

Practice avoiding the use of "why" questions. Revise the questions on the left into a more neutral question or into a statement followed by a more neutral question that asks the client for the same information. The first one has been done for you.

"Why" Question	Transformation
1. "Why didn't you finish breakfast?"	1. "I noticed you didn't finish breakfast. How is your appetite?"
2. "Why are you concerned about your surgery?"	2. ______________________
3. "Why are you feeling anxious?"	3. ______________________
4. "Why didn't you tell the doctor about your symptoms?"	4. ______________________
5. "Why aren't you happy about going home?"	5. ______________________

▶ Activity 4.26: Practice Avoiding "Why" Questions

Review the dialog between the nurse and Ms. Martínez. Write down the examples of "why" questions that you identified. What questions could the nurse have used instead? Write alternative questions that the nurse could have used.

Examples of "Why" Questions	Alternative Questions
______________________	______________________
______________________	______________________
______________________	______________________
______________________	______________________

Culture in Nursing: Cultural Differences in Exploring Personal Health–Related Issues

Some nurses may have difficulty asking clients personal questions about certain topics, such as sexual functioning, alcohol and drug use, and smoking. In many cultures, these topics are taboo; they are considered private matters and are not discussed openly, especially with an elder.

As a result of feeling shy or ashamed to ask personal health–related questions, a nurse may avoid asking these questions altogether or may not ask any follow-up focused or probing questions, even though the client may need help with one of these areas. Rather than showing respect for a client's privacy by not asking personal questions, the nurse's failure to address these areas may have a negative effect on the client's health.

It is, therefore, important that nurses become comfortable asking personal questions and discussing these topics. It is also important that nurses put aside any personal feelings they may have that might prejudice them against a client because of lifestyle differences. Both of these skills can be developed through self-reflection and practice.

▶ Activity 4.27: Considering Cultural Differences in Exploring Personal Health–Related Issues

Determine your answers to the following questions.

1. Are you comfortable discussing personal health–related issues? Why or why not?

___

___

2. Are there some personal health–related issues that are more difficult for you to discuss than others? If so, which ones, and why?

___

___

3. Do you agree with the statement: "Rather than showing respect for a client's privacy by not asking personal questions, the nurse's failure to address these areas may have a negative effect on the client's health?" Why or why not?

___

___

4. What concerns do you have as a nurse in discussing personal health–related issues with a client?

___

___

5. What are some strategies you could use to become more comfortable in asking questions and discussing personal health–related topics with clients?

___

___

Chapter Four Answer Key

Activity 4.1: Addressing Personal Health–Related Issues

1. Ms. Martínez has bulimia nervosa, a type of eating disorder. Eating disorders are a type of mental illness, and both genetic and environmental factors are considered contributing factors to the development of eating disorders. Bulimia nervosa often co-occurs with other psychiatric disorders such as depression, obsessive-compulsive disorder, substance abuse, self-injurious behavior, and anorexia nervosa, another type of eating disorder. (Source: Duckworth, K., and J. L. Freedman. "Bulimia nervosa fact sheet." National Alliance on Mental Illness. Available online. URL: http://www.nami.org/Template.cfm?Section=By_Illness&Template=/ContentManagement/ContentDisplay.cfm&ContentID=149448. Updated January 2013.)

2. Answers will vary, but some knowledge of bulimia nervosa as a type of eating disorder is likely due to media coverage of the issue. Bulimia nervosa is characterized by the rapid consumption of usually unhealthy food, followed by some form of purging, usually self-induced vomiting. Ms. Martínez has been diagnosed with the purging type of bulimia nervosa. People with bulimia nervosa are overly concerned with their body image and engage in patterns of binging and purging in an attempt to control their body weight and shape. (Source: Duckworth, K., and J. L. Freedman. "Bulimia nervosa fact sheet.") Self-induced vomiting can damage parts of the digestive system, including the esophagus and stomach, and cause acid reflux, complications that Ms. Martínez has been diagnosed with.

   Although the exact cause of bulimia is unknown, there are many possible factors that could play a role in the development of an eating disorder, including biological factors, emotional health, and societal expectations. ("Diseases and conditions: Eating disorders." Mayo Clinic. Available online. URL: http://www.mayoclinic.org/diseases-conditions/eating-disorders/basics/causes/con-20033575. Updated on February 8, 2012.) Eating disorders are associated with "unrealistic expectations of slenderness and attractiveness, changes in the role of women, and social standards and attitudes towards obesity." (Shuriquie, N. "Eating disorders: A transcultural perspective." *Eastern Mediterranean Health Journal* 5(1999):2, 354–360.) Eating disorders occur primarily in young white women of middle- and upper-class background. Researchers have found, however, that girls and young women from all ethnic backgrounds, as well as girls with immigrant backgrounds, like Ms. Martínez, are also susceptible to eating disorders, as a function of their exposure to and acceptance of thinness as the new, dominant standard of beauty and the pressure to be thin to be accepted in mainstream American culture.

   Testimony given in support of the Federal Response to Eliminate Eating Disorder Act by Sarah Yeung, an immigrant from Hong Kong, poignantly describes the challenges she faced trying to fit in as an adolescent in the United States:

   > My eating disorder symptoms started when I was 14, a year after my family immigrated to the U.S. from Hong Kong. It was a very difficult transition to American middle school. I felt lost, lonely and out of control. In addition to the usual teenage turmoil, everything I knew became conflicts as my 2 cultures clashed. I wasn't sure what I was supposed to do, how I felt, and ultimately who I was. I spoke with an accent. I looked different. I didn't belong. I didn't fit in. My sense of self was in jeopardy and I became more and more depressed… Similar to many first generation immigrants, I felt great pressure to succeed, to make the sacrifices my parents made to move to the U.S. worthwhile, and to live the 'American dream.' In addition to being biologically predisposed to eating disorders and a history of trauma, the high expectation to achieve culturally and as an immigrant further increased the risk. I felt that I had to be the best at whatever I did. Of course, the trouble with such a standard is that nothing was ever going to be good enough. (Source: Yeung, Sarah. "Remarks for the April 24, 2012, congressional briefing hosted by Senator

Tom Harkin and Eating Disorder Coalition re: Federal response to eliminate Eating Disorder Act." Eating Disorders Coalition. Available online. URL: http://www.eatingdisorderscoalition.org/documents/SarahYeungEDCLobby201204.pdf. Accessed on August 15, 2013.)

3. Because eating disorders are a type of mental illness, a psychiatric consult has been ordered for Ms. Martínez. Although medications are used to treat symptoms of bulimia nervosa, therapy is a cornerstone of treatment for the disorder, including family psychotherapy. However, in many cultures, including in Latino culture, there is a stigma associated with mental illness, which may be why the parents of Ms. Martínez are reluctant to participate in family counseling. Likewise, they may also be reluctant to have their daughter meet with a psychiatrist. (Source: Sanchez, E. L. "Latina struggles when eating disorders and culture collide." NBC Latino. Available online. URL: http://nbclatino.com/2013/02/09/latina-struggles-when-eating-disorders-and-culture-collide/. Posted on February 9, 2009.)

4. In addition to family psychotherapy, group psychotherapy with other Latino adolescents could be helpful, to provide Ms. Martínez with a culturally appropriate environment that is both supportive and therapeutic during the treatment process. Some topics that could be addressed in group therapy include body image in Latino and mainstream U.S. cultures (both traditional and changing); cultural challenges in migration and adaptation to U.S. culture; and strategies to counter societal expectations regarding body image and build self-esteem and body acceptance.

   In addition to group psychotherapy, nutritional counseling could be helpful in guiding Ms. Martínez toward a healthy diet, especially given the easy availability of unhealthy foods in the United States. In addition to a psychiatric consult, a dietician consult has been ordered for Ms. Martínez.

▶ Activity 4.2: Understanding Client Talk—Describing Bodily Functions

Medical/Nursing Term(s)

a. cerumen
b. congestion
c. defecating
d. diaphoretic
e. diarrhea
f. emesis
g. epistaxis
h. eructation
i. flatulence
j. foul body odor
k. halitosis
l. pyrosis
m. mucus
n. nausea
o. perspiration
p. pulse
q. saliva
r. sinus drainage
s. urinating, voiding

Layperson's Term(s)

1. ___k___ bad breath
2. ___m___ snot
3. ___q___ spit
4. ___g___ bloody nose
5. ___s___ peeing
6. ___p___ heartbeat

7. ____o____ sweat
8. ____n____ feeling like you're going to vomit
9. ____r____ runny nose, post-nasal drip
10. ____a____ earwax
11. ____b____ stuffy nose
12. ____c____ pooping
13. ____h____ belching, burping
14. ____e____ the runs
15. ____l____ heartburn
16. ____d____ sweaty
17. ____j____ B.O., smelly
18. ____i____ farting, passing gas
19. ____f____ puke, barf, throw up, vomit

Medical/Nursing Vocabulary

acid reflux: flowing back of secretions from the stomach with an abnormally high concentration of acid

asthma: chronic inflammatory lung disorder marked by recurring and variable episodes of airway obstruction manifested by labored breathing accompanied especially by breathlessness, wheezing and coughing, and a sense of constriction in the chest

bout: sudden attack of a disease, especially one that recurs

bulimia nervosa (purging type): self-imposed eating disorder characterized by weight loss, endocrine dysfunction, and an altered attitude toward weight and eating

dormant: inactive for a period of time

eating disorder: any of several psychological disorders (as anorexia nervosa or bulimia) characterized by serious disturbances of eating behavior

eradicate: kill

flare up: sudden appearance or worsening of symptoms of a disease or condition

fluid: liquid substance that tends to flow or conform to the outline of its container

gastritis: inflammation especially of the mucous membrane of the stomach

gastroesophageal reflux disease (GERD): chronic condition characterized by periodic episodes of gastroesophageal reflux

high Fowler's position: HOB is at a 80–90° angle while the client is lying supine, to prevent GERD after eating

inhibit: prevent

intermittent: not continuous, coming and going at intervals

orally: given or taken through or by way of the mouth

peptic ulcer disease (PUD): erosion of the lining of the stomach or first part of the small intestine, called the duodenum

pernicious anemia: chronic anemia marked by a progressive decrease in number and increase in size and hemoglobin content of red blood cells and by sore, beefy red tongue, pallor, weakness, and gastrointestinal and sensory disturbances, associated with reduced ability to absorb vitamin B12

psychiatric consult: consultation with a doctor specializing in mental disorders

secretion: substance produced by a gland, an organ in the body containing cells that secrete substances that act elsewhere, such as hormones, sweat, or saliva

stool: discharge of fecal matter or feces (feces: bodily waste discharged through the anus)

tarry: having the color of tar, usually stool, caused by hemorrhaging in the stomach or small intestine

triage nurse: nurse who sorts and allocates treatment to clients according to the urgency of their need for care

upright: in a vertical position even when seated at 90°

urine test (or **urinalysis):** lab test that checks the balance of urine components

wheeze: high-pitched or musical whistling sound usually heard on expiration

▶ Activity 4.3: Understanding Medication Orders

1. tetracycline 250 milligrams by mouth 4 times per day
2. furosemide (Lasix) 40 milligrams by mouth immediately
3. ampicillin 500 milligrams intravenous every 6 hours
4. lente insulin 36 units subcutaneous in the morning before meal
5. codeine 30 milligrams by mouth every 4–6 hours as needed for pain
6. atorvastatin (Lipitor) 20 milligrams by mouth every day
7. insulin glargine (Lantus) 10 units subcutaneously every morning
8. 5% dextrose in water intravenous solution 100 mL per hour
9. one dose of ceftriaxone (Rocephin) 500 mg intramuscularly
10. acetaminophen (Tylenol) 120 milligrams rectally every 4 hours as needed for temperature over 102°F

▶ Activity 4.4: Understanding Medications in Scenario #4

Medication		Route	Purpose
1. b	normal saline	IV	a. To reduce fever over 100.2°
2. e	omeprazole	PO	b. To maintain hydration and fluid balance
3. f	famotidine	IV push	c. To eradicate bacteria causing the infection
4. c	amoxicillin	PO	d. To relieve pain
5. d	hydrocodone with acetaminophen	PO	e. To reduce gastric acid secretion
6. a	ibuprofen	PO	f. To inhibit gastric acid secretion, prevent acid-induced inflammation, and promote healing of the ulcer

▶ Activity 4.5: Understanding Nursing Actions in Scenario #4

Nursing Action		Purpose
1. e	maintain on non-irritating diet	a. To monitor vital signs, especially blood pressure, as client is hypotensive
2. d	take daily weight	b. To replenish fluid loss from bleeding and dehydration
3. a	take vitals every 4 hours	c. To decrease acid reflux after eating while assessing cardiovascular status
4. g	check O_2 sats every 4 hours	d. To monitor for weight loss because of client's eating disorder
5. f	contact clinician if O_2 sats fall below 90%	e. To treat peptic ulcer
6. b	encourage fluids orally	f. To request new orders for client, as needed
7. c	after eating, maintain client upright or elevate HOB at 90° for 3 hours and monitor vital signs every 15 minutes	g. To monitor for oxygen loss due to bleeding and dehydration

▶ Activity 4.6: Plan of Care: Planning for Client's Care

1. PUD (peptic ulcer disease)
2. Bulimia nervosa (purging type), gastritis, asthma, intermittent GERD, pernicious anemia
3. Hydrocodone with acetaminophen (Vicodin); 10 mg; every 4–6 hours, as needed
4. Omeprazole and amoxicillin at 8:00 a.m. and 8:00 p.m.; 20 mg omeprazole, 1,000 mg amoxicillin
5. Labs: urine test, CBC; Appts: psychiatric and dietician consults
6. High Fowler's position (90°) for 3 hours after meals.

Nursing Diagnosis: Planning Holistic Care for Ms. Martínez

"Nurse will teach the client importance of adequate nutritional intake and the consequences of purging by discharge date" reflects holistic care of Ms. Martínez's eating disorder. It addresses Ms. Martínez's psychosocial needs by educating her about eating disorders.

▶ Activity 4.7: Nursing Diagnosis: Desired Outcomes and Nursing Interventions

Nursing Intervention	Desired Outcome
1. __d__ Nurse will administer GI medication and analgesics and monitor for side effects during shift.	a. Blood pressure will be 120/80 mmHg by the end of shift.
2. __b__ Nurse will monitor vital signs, lab values, and signs of GI bleeding closely throughout shift.	b. Hemoglobin and hematocrit will be within normal limits within 48 hours.
3. __a__ Nurse will monitor fluid input and output closely throughout shift.	c. Client will describe expected daily dietary intake and adverse effects of purging by time of discharge.
4. __c__ Nurse will teach client the importance of adequate nutritional intake and the consequences of purging by discharge date.	d. Client will report pain level of 3 (scale 0–10) and decreased anxiety within 1 hour of analgesic administration.

▶ Activity 4.8: Understanding Nursing Diagnoses and Goals

Nursing Diagnosis	Goal
1. __h__ Caregiver role strain	a. Express spiritual well-being
2. __f__ Interrupted family processes	b. Improved communication
3. __g__ Dysfunctional grieving	c. Healthy self-concept
4. __b__ Impaired verbal communication	d. Experience control
5. __i__ Ineffective coping	e. Diminished pain
6. __c__ Disturbed body image	f. Improve family process
7. __e__ Acute pain	g. Grieve appropriately
8. __j__ Ineffective breastfeeding	h. Adequate role performance
9. __a__ Readiness for enhanced spiritual well-being	i. Effective coping
10. __d__ Powerlessness	j. Effective breastfeeding

▶ Activity 4.9: Matching Nursing Diagnoses and Goals

Nursing Diagnosis	Goal
1. __c__ Impaired skin integrity	a. Adequate fluid volume
2. __d__ Impaired spontaneous ventilation	b. Decrease in pain
3. __b__ Acute pain	c. Improved skin integrity
4. __a__ Deficient fluid volume	d. Adequate energy level and muscle function to maintain spontaneous breathing

▶ Activity 4.10: Understanding the Language of Desired Outcomes

Desired Outcome–Vague Wording	Desired Outcome–Specific Wording
1. __h__ less pain	a. will report absence of nausea throughout day shift
2. __j__ feel rested	b. will use 2 or fewer ABD dressings to incision site per 8-hour shift
3. __e__ understand better	c. will have urine output of at least 30 mL/hr for 8-hour period
4. __a__ less nausea	d. will attend all therapy sessions
5. __c__ adequate voiding	e. will verbalize understanding of discharge instructions
6. __g__ less anxious	f. will identify at least 3 factors that can be controlled by client
7. __b__ less drainage	g. will demonstrate one or more relaxation techniques before invasive procedure
8. __i__ increased appetite	h. will rate pain 3 or less on scale of 0–10
9. __f__ experience increased sense of control	i. will consume at least 70% of all meals
10. __d__ participate in activities	j. will have at least 4 hours of uninterrupted sleep at night

Activity 4.11: Understanding Nursing Interventions

1. Monitor for verbalization of help needed to use commode after every meal.
2. Instruct client to avoid drinking alcohol while on medication.
3. Raise the head of bed during periods of shortness of breath.
4. Discuss with client and spouse cancer support group resources before discharge.
5. Palpate abdomen for tenderness once during shift.
6. Teach Kegel exercises to prevent urinary incontinence while sneezing, coughing, or laughing before the end of shift.
7. Demonstrate blood pressure assessment technique once and repeat as needed.
8. Monitor blood glucose testing skills every shift.
9. Assess newly inserted gastric tube site for S/S of infection every 8 hours.
10. Reposition client every 2 hours.

Activity 4.12: Understanding Telephone Report

1. The vomiting in Scenario #4 is due to internal bleeding in the abdomen from PUD. The vomiting in the telephone report is due to purging after eating (as a manifestation of bulimia nervosa). The immediate cause of vomiting is different in the 2 instances, but they are related in the sense that Ms. Martínez has PUD because of bulimia nervosa.
2. Dark and tarry stools indicate gastrointestinal bleeding from PUD.
3. The amount of oxygen in the client's blood has decreased due to the bleeding. There are fewer red cells available to carry the oxygen to the body.
4. The client's BP initially increased due to the NS IV, which hydrates the client and balances the electrolytes. However, the client continues to experience gastric hemorrhaging (or bleeding in the stomach), once again reducing her BP.

Activity 4.13: Understanding Telephone Order

1. Ferrous sulfate, to boost the client's iron, oral drops
2. 10 mg (in telephone order); 10 mg (in Scenario #4). No difference in amount of medication, but frequency of administration has changed. In telephone order frequency is every 4 hours, and in Scenario #4 frequency is every 4–6 hours PRN. The new medication order (with the greater frequency of administration) is in response to the client's intense stomach pain.
3. Esomeprazole (Nexium), 80 mg (in telephone order), once.
4. Every 4–6 hours, to decrease wheezing, through inhaler, 2 puffs
5. 0.9% NS 150 mL per hour (in telephone order) compared to 0.9% NS 100 mL per hour in Scenario #4. The flow rate has been increased to more effectively improve hydration and promote fluid balance in the client.

6. The telephone order calls for Ms. Martínez's blood pressure to be checked every 15 minutes for 12 hours. In Scenario #4, the blood pressure was checked as part of the vital signs every 4 hours except after meals, when it was checked every 15 minutes for 3 hours. The client is hypotensive but is positioned upright for 3 hours after meals to avoid acid reflux. Because there is continued bleeding and a BP drop from 118/77 mm Hg (in the Plan of Care) to 97/60 mm Hg (in the telephone report), BP is checked every 15 minutes for the next 12 hours, rather than just the 3 hours after meals.

▶ Activity 4.14: Addressing Personal Health–Related Issues

1. Three of the 4 nursing interventions address physiological consequences of bulimia nervosa (purging type): GI bleeding from peptic ulcer disease and gastritis; dehydration from the bleeding; and stomach pain. In addition to addressing the immediate physiological needs of the client, one nursing intervention addresses the psychosocial dimension of eating disorders by emphasizing the role of educating the client about the disorder. By addressing both the client's physiological as well as psychosocial needs, the nursing interventions reflect holistic care of the client. However, before addressing the client's psychosocial needs, the nurse needs to first take care of the client's physiological needs.

2. During the client's unstable period, she vomited bloody vomitus and was wheezing; her stool was dark and tarry; she experienced intense stomach pain; she was pale and weak; her bowel sounds were hyperactive; her O_2 sats dropped; and her BP decreased.

3. All aspects of the plan (of care) in the progress note address the client's eating disorder, at least indirectly. For example, teaching client the importance of keeping the head of bed (HOB) upright at least 3 hours after meals is to prevent the reoccurrence of GERD (gastroesophageal reflux disease), one consequence of bulimia nervosa (purging type). Because of the dehydration caused by the GI bleeding that the client is experiencing as a result of having PUD (peptic ulcer disease)–another consequence of bulimia nervosa (purging type)–the client is supposed to drink lots of fluids. In addition, the client's health status and progress continues to be monitored and medications administered per MAR. These aspects of the plan (of care) address the client's physiological needs, but the client has psychosocial needs related to her eating disorder, as well. To promote the client's psychological well-being and thus provide holistic care, the nurse provides a quiet, healing environment. The nurse encourages the client to eat progressively more food and to avoid purging, thus providing the psychological support for the changes in behavior that are necessary to resolving peptic ulcer disease. To establish a relationship of trust, an important aspect of holistic care, the nurse discusses the plan of care with the client and her family and encourages the client to talk with the nurse about any concerns she has regarding her health and care. The client also agrees to see an eating disorder therapist.

4. The plan (of care) in the progress note recognizes the importance of family in many cultures by including the family in the discussion of the client's care. However, later in the dialog, the nurse offers to refer the client to an eating disorder therapist without letting the parents know. (See answer to question #6 in Activity 4.16 for discussion of the importance of providing confidential care to adolescents.) By providing confidential care to Ms. Martínez, the nurse acknowledges some of the challenges that adolescents face growing up in the United States, particularly those from cultural backgrounds that give priority to family concerns over the individual's concerns.

   Otherwise, there is no discussion in the plan (of care) of culturally sensitive strategies to address Ms. Martínez's eating disorders, besides encouraging the client to discuss any concerns she has with the nurse about her health and care. Depending on the level of trust that is established between the client and nurse, it might be helpful to encourage the client to discuss more specifically any body image concerns she might have, especially differences between Latino and mainstream U.S. cultures (both traditional and changing); cultural challenges in migration and adaptation to U.S. culture; and strategies to counter societal expectations regarding body image and to build self-esteem and body acceptance.

▶ Activity 4.15: Analyzing and Evaluating Documentation

1. Regarding the formatting of the documentation, no date is provided for each entry, and the times provided are not precise. The 24-hour clock is not used; do these times represent a.m. or p.m.? The nurse has not drawn a line through blank space to the end of the line, to prevent someone else from adding to the documentation at a later time. The nurse has neither signed his or her name nor provided a title.

   Regarding conciseness, the nurse has written complete sentences rather than thought units ("She complains of pain in her knees.) The nurse has not used abbreviations ("pt" instead of "patient" and "c/o" instead of "complains of"). The nurse has included words that do not carry meaning ("to take a" and "the").

   Regarding objectivity, the nurse uses the word "worrier," which implies disapproval of the client. "No success" also implies a negative judgment of the client.

   Regarding completeness, the nurse has not provided complete information. First, what did the nurse discuss with the client? Was that information helpful in caring for the client? Second, 2 different BPs are listed, but T is not included. What is the client's temperature? Were the 2 BPs taken in different positions or at different times? Third, no information is provided regarding why the client refused to take a bath. Fourth, the nurse assumes that the client fell in the bathroom. What evidence is there that she fell? Did the nurse walk in and see the client on the floor, or did the client report that she fell? Are there any bruises on the client as a result of the fall?

   Regarding precision, the nurse has not provided precise information. Instead of "for a while," the nurse should state exactly how long the nurse and client talked. The nurse should provide a more precise description of the client's pain. On a scale of 0–10, how does the client rate her pain? What words does the client use to describe her pain? Is it constant or intermittent? Does it radiate to other parts of her body?

2. The nurse should use the nursing process as a framework for documentation: assessment, diagnosis, planning, implementation, evaluation. Assessment findings that relate to *Impaired physical mobility related to stiffness* should be documented, including objective and subjective data. A goal should be included that indicates a healthy response to impaired physical mobility. Nursing actions and interventions that were done to help relieve the stiffness and pain should be documented, as well as the client's response to those interventions, or outcomes. In addition, any teaching that was done and the client's response should be documented.

The following statements relate to questions 3–6:

a. "I couldn't sleep at all last night"
b. Positioned supine with pillow behind head
c. Muscle relaxant relieves stiffness in knees
d. Pt rated pain at 6 on a scale of 0 to 10
e. "I can move my knees more easily now" (after interventions)
f. Muscle relaxant administered 2 hours ago
g. Warm pack placed around knees
h. BP 128/87 P 75 RR 16
i. Give muscle relaxant around the clock q6h versus q8h
j. "Dull, constant pain in knees that radiates to thighs"
k. Rubs knees constantly
l. Pt rated pain at 3 on a scale of 0 to 10
m. Perform passive ROM exercises to legs, as tolerated

3. Which statement(s) represent subjective data? a, d, j
4. Which statement(s) represent objective data? h, k
5. Which statement(s) represent nursing actions and interventions? b, f, g, i, m
6. Which statement(s) represent outcomes? c, e, l

Activity 4.16: Analyzing Effectiveness of Communication

1. Answers will vary, but there are at least 5 examples of ineffective interviewing techniques in the interview, as follows:

   - The nurse does not ask an open-ended question at the beginning of the interview (e.g., How are you feeling?), but rather asks several focused questions about eating, one right after the other: "What have you been eating this past month? How much do you eat at one time? How often do you eat?" In addition to overwhelming the client and not allowing the client time to answer each of these questions individually, the nurse does not allow the client to talk first about what might be of concern to her. In addition to an open-ended question at the beginning of the interview, it would be helpful for the nurse to provide a transition into the topic of the interview: Ms. Martínez's eating habits, such as, "I want to talk with you about your eating habits."
   - Toward the beginning of the interview, Ms. Martínez lists the kinds of foods that she likes to eat. The foods are mostly unhealthy fast foods like pizza and chicken tenders. The nurse then asks, "Why do you eat these foods?" In response to this question, Ms. Martínez starts to get defensive. Her intonation rises and there is a negative tone in her voice when she responds, "What do you mean…? I just like to eat them!"
   - Ms. Martínez is clearly uncomfortable when she first begins talking about purging. Rather than the nurse using therapeutic communication techniques, such as reflecting implied feelings, providing nonverbal reassurance, and remaining silent, the nurse asks, "Why won't you tell me?" and then states, "I care about your well-being." Although the second statement could have been an effective use of "I" statement and could have provided verbal reassurance, here it seems to place added pressure on Ms. Martínez to give the nurse the information that she wants. In response to this question, Ms. Martínez gets defensive and states, "Because people will judge me, and I kind of feel that way right now."
   - When Ms. Martínez is talking about purging, she begins to cry. Rather than the nurse using therapeutic communication techniques–such as reflecting feelings, providing nonverbal reassurance, and remaining silent–the nurse asks, "Why do you make yourself vomit after you eat?" In response to this question, Ms. Martínez replies, "I don't know," and looks away.
   - After the discussion of eating habits, the nurse begins asking a series of closed questions: "Do you have friends at school?" "Are you dating anyone?" "How is your relationship with your parents?" Although the nurse asks these questions one at a time, they are closed questions, resulting in very brief responses from Ms. Martínez: "A few," "No," and "It's okay," respectively.

2. In addition to the effect of each individual instance of ineffective communication, as discussed in the answer to #1, the overall effect is generally a tense and unhappy atmosphere at times during the interview. Ms. Martínez responds defensively several times and stops talking at other times. In addition, she does not provide meaningful responses to the nurse's questions until the end of the interview, thus prolonging the interview unnecessarily.

3. Eventually, the nurse is able to gather some information about Ms. Martínez's personal health–related issues, but not without potentially damaging the relationship of trust between the nurse and client and limiting the therapeutic benefits of the interview. Although the client's responses to some of the

initial questions about school, friends, and a significant other are minimal, Ms. Martínez does open up and talk about feeling lonely, different, and ignored while also wanting to fit in and be like everyone else, including having the same body type as others (tall and thin with blonde hair). Such information could help the nurse address the root causes of Ms. Martínez's eating disorder.

4. Overall, the interview is not an example of therapeutic communication because the nurse missed so many opportunities to use therapeutic communication techniques, as discussed in #1: reflecting feelings (both stated and implied), providing nonverbal reassurance, and remaining silent. In addition, the nurse used several examples of pitfalls to effective interviewing, especially the use of "why" questions, which can be perceived as judging the client or expressing disapproval, both of which are blocks to therapeutic communication.

5. The nurse could use more therapeutic communication skills in her interaction with Ms. Martínez. In addition to specific skills, such as those mentioned in #1 (reflecting feelings, providing nonverbal reassurance, and remaining silent), the nurse could show greater empathy toward the client and attend to the client more effectively. Also, the nurse could use more effective interviewing techniques, in particular open-ended questions.

6. Answers will vary, but according to Advocates for Youth, providing confidential health services is essential to promoting and providing health care to adolescents, especially services related to sexual and reproductive health, drug and alcohol use, and mental health. (Source: Loxterman, J. "Adolescent access to confidential health services." Advocates for Youth. Available online. URL: http://www.advocatesforyouth.org/component/content/article/516-adolescent-access-to-confidential-health-services. Posted July 1997.) Such confidentiality is more important than including parents in the decision-making process, as many adolescents will not seek preventative care or treatment for personal health–related issues if they think their parents will be informed. For example, one study found that only 45% of adolescents would seek care for depression if parental notification were required. Confidentiality is also important for health care providers. Adolescents may not reveal sensitive but relevant information to health care providers if they fear such information will not be kept private. However, without such information, health care providers may not be able to determine an accurate diagnosis and provide appropriate treatment.

   Because parental notification may discourage adolescents from seeking the care they need, which could have negative health implications not only for adolescents but also for others around them, many states have laws that protect teen confidentiality for specific services, especially related to reproductive and sexual health, drug and alcohol treatment, and mental health. Adolescents are at a critical stage of development, both physically and emotionally. They are also beginning to establish their own identity and autonomy. Teens experiencing serious health issues, such as sexually transmitted diseases (STDs), pregnancy, sexual abuse, depression, rage, or suicidal thoughts, may endanger themselves and those around them. Protecting their confidentiality encourages adolescents to seek the care they need and allows health care providers to deliver the necessary care.

   Although this perspective may be difficult to understand and accept for students from cultures where the family, not the individual, is the locus of decision-making, it is important to understand the values that are at play in the U.S. health care context: that is, the principle of beneficence, or "doing good" for the client, as well as individual autonomy, or the right of individuals to know their health status and to make their own decisions with regard to their health care. Furthermore, there is legal authority behind these values, as states have determined that protecting confidentiality for adolescents is more important than promoting parental control and family autonomy in situations where parental notification might deter adolescents from seeking essential health services.

   Therefore, in the situation of Ms. Martínez seeking mental health counseling for her eating disorder, the nurse is not obligated to inform the parents or to include them in the decision-making process.

▶ Activity 4.17: Analyzing Dialog for Personal Questions

In addition to asking Ms. Martínez about her eating disorder, the nurse asks several questions about other personal health–related issues: "Do you have friends at school?" "Are you dating anyone?" "Do you drink alcohol or take drugs?" and "Do you have a good relationship with your parents?" Although Ms. Martínez does not have a boyfriend, drink alcohol, or take drugs, her response, both verbal and nonverbal (she looks away and her eyes begin to water), to the question whether she has any friends prompts the nurse to ask an open-ended follow-up question: "Tell me about school" followed by a closed question: "Are you happy in your school?" Ms. Martínez's extended response about her challenges trying to fit in and her feelings about being different reveals the source of her disturbed body image, information that should be very helpful for the nurse.

▶ Activity 4.18: Analyzing Dialog for Multiple Questions

There is one example of the use of multiple questions. At the beginning of the interview, the nurse asks several focused questions about eating, all at one time–"What have you been eating this past month? How much do you eat at one time? How often do you eat?"–rather than asking an open-ended question. In addition to overwhelming the client and not allowing the client time to answer each of these questions individually, the nurse does not allow the client to talk first about what might be of concern to her. Thus, any therapeutic benefits of the interaction between the nurse and client are not realized.

▶ Activity 4.19: Transforming Multiple Questions

Multiple Questions	Transformation
1. "How do you feel this morning–did you get enough sleep last night and enough to eat for breakfast?"	1. "How do you feel this morning?" (pause for reply) "How did you sleep last night?" (pause for reply) "How was breakfast?" (pause for reply)
2. "Where do you live, how many people live with you, and who do you live with?"	2. "Tell me about your living situation."
3. "Did stress, diet, exercise, or something else cause the problem?"	3. "What do you think caused the problem?"

▶ Activity 4.20: Practice Avoiding Multiple Questions

Examples of Multiple Questions	Alternative Questions
"What have you been eating this past month? How much do you eat at one time? How often do you eat?"	"Tell me about your eating habits this past month."

▶ Activity 4.21: Analyzing Dialog for Closed Questions

After the discussion of Ms. Martínez's eating habits, the nurse asks a series of closed questions: "Do you have friends at school?" "Are you dating anyone?" and "How is your relationship with your parents?" Although the nurse asks these questions one at a time, they are closed questions, resulting in very brief responses from Ms. Martínez: "A few," "No," and "It's okay," respectively. It's only when the nurse begins asking open-ended questions: "Tell me about school" (although this question has to be clarified with a follow-up focused question that is closed: "Are you happy in your school?"), followed by an open-ended probe: "Tell me more," that the client begins to open up and talk about issues of concern to her.

▶ Activity 4.22: Transforming Closed Questions

Closed Questions	Open-Ended Questions
1. "Are you feeling pain?"	1. "Tell me about the pain."
2. "Are you taking any medication?"	2. "What medications are you taking?"
3. "Are you available at 11 o'clock for your next appointment?"	3. "When are you available for your next appointment?"
4. "Are you exercising regularly?"	4. "Tell me about your physical activity."
5. "How often do you exercise?"	5. "What kinds of exercises do you do?"

▶ Activity 4.23: Practice Avoiding Closed Questions

Examples of Closed Questions	Alternative Questions
"Do you have friends at school?"	"Tell me about your friendships at school."
"Are you dating anyone?"	"If you are dating someone, how do you spend your time together?"
"Do you have a good relationship with your parents?"	"How is your relationship with your parents?"

▶ Activity 4.24: Analyzing Dialog for "Why" Questions

There are 3 examples of "why" questions in the interview.

Toward the beginning of the interview, Ms. Martínez lists the kinds of foods that she likes to eat. The foods are mostly unhealthy fast foods like pizza and chicken tenders. The nurse then asks: "Why do you eat these foods?" In response to this "why" question, Ms. Martínez gets defensive. Her intonation rises and she responds with a negative tone in her voice: "What do you mean…? I just like to eat them!"

A little later in the interview, Ms. Martínez is clearly uncomfortable when she first begins talking about purging. Rather than the nurse using therapeutic communication techniques, such as reflecting implied feelings, providing nonverbal reassurance, and remaining silent, the nurse asks, "Why won't you tell me?" The use of a "why" question here comes across as judgmental. In response, Ms. Martínez gets defensive and replies, "Because people will judge me, and I kind of feel that way right now."

Later, when Ms. Martínez is talking about purging, she begins to cry. Rather than the nurse using therapeutic communication techniques (reflecting, providing nonverbal reassurance, and remaining silent), the nurse asks, "Why do you make yourself vomit after you eat?" Again, the use of a "why" question here comes across as judgmental. Ms. Martínez responds by essentially shutting down. She replies, "I don't know," and looks away.

▶ Activity 4.25: Transforming "Why" Questions

"Why" Question	Transformation
1. "Why didn't you finish breakfast?"	1. "I noticed you didn't finish breakfast. How is your appetite?"
2. "Why are you concerned about your surgery?"	2. "You seem concerned about your surgery today. Do you have any questions that I can help you with?"
3. "Why are you feeling anxious?"	3. "You seem anxious. Has something happened?"
4. "Why didn't you tell the doctor about your symptoms?"	4. "What prevented you from coming to the clinic earlier?"
5. "Why aren't you happy about going home?"	5. "Tell me more about how you're feeling."

▶ Activity 4.26: Practice Avoiding "Why" Questions

Examples of "Why" Questions	Alternative Questions
"Why do you eat these foods?"	"What about these foods do you like?"
"Why won't you tell me?"	"Tell me what you're concerned about."
"Why do you make yourself vomit after you eat?"	"What makes you want to throw up after you eat?"

▶ Activity 4.27: Considering Cultural Differences in Exploring Personal Health–Related Issues

1–4: Answers will vary.

5. Reading articles about personal health–related topics and discussing them with friends, family, co-workers, and supervisors could help prepare you to ask questions about these topics with clients. Similarly, discussion with U.S. co-workers and friends about cultural differences in personal health–related issues could also help you to become more comfortable discussing these topics with clients.

APPENDIX: Medical/Nursing Abbreviations

(+) positive

° degree

Abd abdominal

AC before meals

ADLs activities of daily living

BG blood glucose

BID twice a day

BP blood pressure

BUN blood urea nitrogen

CAM complementary and alternative medicine

CBC complete blood count

c/o complain(ed) of

COPD chronic obstructive pulmonary disease

D_5W 5% dextrose in water

D/C discontinue(d)

DJD degenerative joint disease

dL deciliter

DM diabetes mellitus

DNR/DNI do not resuscitate/do not intubate

drsg dressing

Dx diagnosis

ECG electrocardiogram

fld fluid

g gram

GERD gastroesophageal reflux disease

HOB head of bed

h hour

hr hour

HTN hypertension

I&O input and output (refers to a client's fluid status, specifically fluid intake and urine output, usually within a 24-hour period)

IM intramuscular injection

IV intravenous

IVP intravenous pyelogram

IVPB IV piggyback (Intravenous piggyback is delivery of medication that is continuous or by drip)

IV push IV delivery of medication that is pushed in as scheduled; IV push is delivery of medication that is intermittent.

JVD jugular venous distention

L liter

Ⓛ left (When L means "left," it is circled to avoid confusion with other abbreviations (such as L for "liter.")

LPN/LVN licensed practical nurse/licensed vocational nurse

MAR medication administration record

mcg microgram

MD medical doctor

med/surg medical/surgical

meds medications

mg milligram

MHx medical history

MI myocardial infarction

min minute(s)

mL milliliter

Na^+ sodium

NAP nursing assistive personnel

NC nasal cannula

NKA no known allergies

NPH neutral protamine Hagedorn, a type of insulin that is intermediate flow and long-lasting (24 hours' duration)

NPO nothing by mouth

NS normal saline

O_2 oxygen

O_2 sats oxygen saturation (also abbreviated SaO_2)

P pulse

PB piggyback

PO by mouth

PRN as needed

pt patient

PUD peptic ulcer disease

q3h every 3 hours (Note: The abbreviation *q* is not used alone, only as part of a time interval.)

q4–6hr every 4–6 hours

Ⓡ right (When R is used to mean "right," it is circled to avoid confusion with other abbreviations, such as R for "respiratory.")

RA rheumatoid arthritis

RA room air

ROM range of motion

RR respiration rate

RRT rapid response team

RT respiratory therapist

SOB short of breath

SSI sliding scale insulin

stat immediately

subcut subcutaneous (under the skin)

T temperature

TID 3 times a day

UTI urinary tract infection

vitals vital signs

VS vital signs

VSS vital signs stable

yo years old